Surgical Pathology of the Head and Neck

Surgical Pathology of the Head and Neck

Dale H. Rice, M.D.
Tiber/Alpert Professor and Chair
Department of Otolaryngology-Head and Neck Surgery
University of Southern California School of Medicine
Los Angeles, California

John G. Batsakis, M.D.
Professor Emeritus, Pathology
Former Chairman, Pathology
University of Texas M.D. Anderson Cancer Center
Houston, Texas

LIPPINCOTT WILLIAMS & WILKINS
A **Wolters Kluwer** Company
Philadelphia · Baltimore · New York · London
Buenos Aires · Hong Kong · Sydney · Tokyo

Acquisitions Editor: Danette Knopp
Developmental Editor: Sara Lauber
Production Editor: Jodi Borgenicht
Manufacturing Manager: Tim Reynolds
Cover Designer: Karen Quigley
Compositor: Maryland Composition

© 2000 by LIPPINCOTT WILLIAMS & WILKINS
227 East Washington Square
Philadelphia, PA 19106-3780 USA
LWW.com

All rights reserved. This book is protected by copyright. No part of this book may be reproduced in any form or by any means, including photocopying, or utilized by any information storage and retrieval system without written permission from the copyright owner, except for brief quotations embodied in critical articles and reviews. Materials appearing in this book prepared by individuals as part of their official duties as U.S. government employees are not covered by the above-mentioned copyright.

Printed in China

Library of Congress Cataloging-in-Publication Data

Rice, Dale H.
    Surgical pathology of the head and neck / Dale H. Rice, John Batsakis.
      p.   cm.
    Includes bibliographical references and index.
    ISBN 0-7817-2354-X
    1. Head—Diseases—Diagnosis.   2. Neck—Diseases—Diagnosis.
3. Pathology, Surgical.   I. Rice, Dale H.   II. Title.
    [DNLM: 1. Head and Neck Neoplasms—pathology.   2. Head and Neck
Neoplasms—surgery.   WE 707 B334s 1999]
RC936.B38   1999
616.99′291—dc21
DNLM/DLC
for Library of Congress   99-35712
                                                                               CIP

Care has been taken to confirm the accuracy of the information presented and to describe generally accepted practices. However, the authors and publisher are not responsible for errors or omissions or for any consequences from application of the information in this book and make no warranty, expressed or implied, with respect to the currency, completeness, or accuracy of the contents of the publication. Application of this information in a particular situation remains the professional responsibility of the practitioner.

The authors and publisher have exerted every effort to ensure that drug selection and dosage set forth in this text are in accordance with current recommendations and practice at the time of publication. However, in view of ongoing research, changes in government regulations, and the constant flow of information relating to drug therapy and drug reactions, the reader is urged to check the package insert for each drug for any change in indications and dosage and for added warnings and precautions. This is particularly important when the recommended agent is a new or infrequently employed drug.

Some drugs and medical devices presented in this publication have Food and Drug Administration (FDA) clearance for limited use in restricted research settings. It is the responsibility of the health care provider to ascertain the FDA status of each drug or device planned for use in their clinical practice.

10 9 8 7 6 5 4 3 2 1

To the faculty and residents of the Department of Otolaryngology—Head and Neck Surgery of the University of Southern California School of Medicine who have taught me so much over the years.

DHR

To my wife, Mary.

JGB

Contents

Preface	xi
Acknowledgments	xii

Part One: Site-Specific Diseases

1 Salivary Glands 3
   Presentation 4
   Pathophysiology 4
   Histogenesis of Salivary Gland Tumors 4
   Histology of Benign Tumors 6
      Pleomorphic Adenoma · Warthin's Tumor
      · Monomorphic Adenomas · Inverted Ductal
      Papilloma · Myoepithelioma · Dermal Analogue
      Tumor Monomorphic Adenoma · Sialoblastoma
      · Sebaceous Tumors
   Histology of Malignant Tumors 20
      General Remarks · Mucoepidermoid Carcinoma
      · Acinic Cell Adenocarcinoma · Malignant Mixed
      Tumor · Adenoid Cystic Carcinoma · Polymorphous
      Low-grade Adenocarcinoma (Terminal Duct
      Adenocarcinoma) · Epimyoepithelial Carcinoma
      · Salivary Duct Carcinoma
   Histology of Nonneoplastic Lesions 36
      Lymphoepithelial Lesions, Sialosis · Sjögren's
      Syndrome · Mucocele/Ranula · Necrotizing
      Sialometaplasia; Sialolithiasis · Sialadenitis

2 Thyroid Gland 47
   Thyroglossal Duct Cyst 48
   Hashimoto's Thyroiditis 48

Graves' Disease 48
Multinodular Goiter 48
Papillary Thyroid Carcinoma 50
Follicular Carcinoma 52
Follicular Variant of Papillary Carcinoma 54
Hürthle Cell Carcinoma 54
Medullary Carcinoma 56
Anaplastic Carcinoma 56

3 Parathyroid Gland 59
Hyperparathyroidism 60
Parathyroid Carcinoma 60

4 Ear 63
Ceruminoma 64
Cholesteatoma 64
Cholesterol Granuloma 64
Malignant External Otitis (Necrotizing External Otitis) 66
Acute Otitis Media 66
Eosinophilic Granuloma 68
Endolymphatic Sac Tumors 68

5 Larynx 71
Vocal Fold Nodules 72
Contact Granulomas and Ulcers 72
Squamous Papilloma 72

6 Sinonasal 75
Nasal Polyps 76
Allergic Fungal Sinusitis 78
Mucormycosis 78
Myospherulosis 80
Wegener's Granulomatosis 80
Inverted Papilloma 82
Fungiform Papilloma 82
Angiofibroma 82
Adenocarcinomas 84
Olfactory Neuroblastoma 86

7 Skin and Fibrous Tissue 89
Junctional Nevus 90
Compound Nevus 90
Intradermal Nevus 90
Actinic Keratosis 90
Seborrheic Keratosis 92
Fibrous Tumors 92
   Fibromatosis · Keloids · Fibrosarcoma · Dermatofibrosarcoma
Melanoma 98
Herpes 98
Candidiasis 98

8	Dental and Bone	103
	Ameloblastoma	104
	Odontogenic Keratocyst	104
	Pindborg Tumor (Calcifying Epithelial Odontogenic Tumor)	106
	Adenomatoid Odontogenic Tumor	106
	Squamous Odontogenic Tumor	106
	Odontogenic Fibroma	108
	Odontogenic Myxoma	108
	Fibrous Dysplasia	110
	Osteoid Osteoma and Osteoblastoma	110
	Ossifying Fibroma	112
	Aneurysmal Bone Cyst	114
	Giant Cell (Reparative) Granuloma	114
	Myxoma	114
	Osteoma	116
	Osteochondroma	116
	Osteosarcoma	118
	Chondroma and Other Cartilage Tumors	120
	Chondrosarcoma	122
	Chordoma	124
	Paget's Disease	124

Part Two: Non-Site Specific Diseases

9	Inflammatory Lesions	129
	Myobacterial Infections	130
	Cat-Scratch Disease	130
	Rhinoscleroma (Scleroma)	130
	Rhinosporidiosis	132
	Leprosy	132
	Blastomycosis	132
	Toxoplasmosis	134
	Coccidioidomycosis	134
	Sarcoidosis	134
10	Benign Neoplasms	137
	Granular Cell Tumor	138
	Schwannoma and Neurofibroma	138
	Lipoma and Hibernoma	140
	Rhabdomyoma	140
	Leiomyoma	140
	Paraganglioma	142
11	Malignant Neoplasms	145
	Squamous Cell Carcinoma	146
	Squamous Cell Carcinoma Variants	150
	Rhabdomyosarcoma	156

	Lymphoma	158
	Plasmacytoma	158
	Leiomyosarcoma	162
	Liposarcoma	162
	Neurosarcoma	162
12	Noninflammatory, Nonneoplastic Diseases	165
	Fordyce's Granules	166
	Amyloidosis	166
	Hemangioma	168
	Lymphangioma	168
	Branchial Cleft Cyst	170
	Nodular Fasciitis	172

Subject Index 175

Preface

This book was written for students interested in pathology of the head and neck, both neoplastic and nonneoplastic. The book is structured to be user-friendly. As much as possible, the organization is such that the text is on the left hand page while the illustrations and legends are on the facing right hand page.

This book is divided into two main sections. The first section covers specific anatomic areas and the diseases associated with those areas, such as the salivary gland. The second section is concerned with diseases that can occur in a wide variety of locations. The most obvious example of the latter is squamous cell carcinoma. In some instances an arbitrary placement was used.

Although not every clinicopathologic entity has been covered, we have attempted to include a large and diverse group of entities. Very little of the content has been expended in covering pathophysiology or treatment, as this book is designed to be neither a pathology treatise nor a textbook on diseases of the head and neck, but rather a color atlas. We hope the study of this book will allow the student to recognize classic disease patterns as they appear in histologic preparations.

Acknowledgments

This book would never have seen the "light of day" without the continual encouragement of Kathey Alexander and Danette Knopp. More proximal help came from Sara Lauber, who enabled the completion of this project.

PART I

Site-specific Diseases

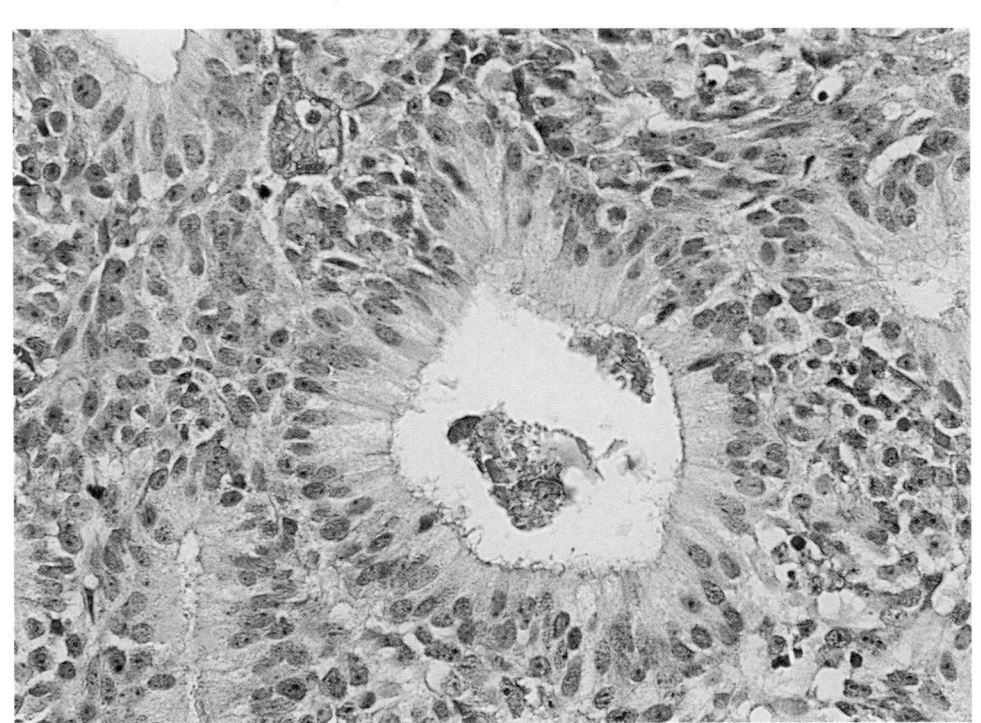

1

Salivary Glands

PRESENTATION

The majority of salivary gland neoplasms present as asymptomatic masses.

PATHOPHYSIOLOGY

The major salivary glands are composed of predominantly serous and mucous glands arranged in lobular units and interconnected by a complex system of excretory ducts. Also present are occasional sebaceous glands. The lobules contain variable amounts of fat. Generally, the amount of fat and number of serous elements are greatest in the major glands and decrease in quantity as the gland decreases in size. Alternatively, the number of mucous cells increases. Lymph nodes within the parotid gland are common and frequently contain salivary gland tissue. Hence, the parotid gland is rich in both serous and fatty elements, with few mucous cells. The submandibular gland contains less fat and more mucous cells, but serous acinar elements still predominate. Lymph nodes are extraparenchymal. The sublingual gland has few serous cells and numerous mucous cells. The intraoral salivary glands are composed almost entirely of mucous elements.

The serous and mucous acini empty into the proximal aspect of the salivary duct system, known as the intercalated duct. Located at the periphery of the acinar unit and intercalated duct are myoepithelial cells, which are thought to have a contractile function. Interposed between the epithelial cells of the intercalated duct are occasional smaller, round hyperchromatic cells known alternatively as basal cells or reserve cells. The intercalated duct becomes the striated duct more distally, then empties into the larger excretory duct, which eventually communicates with the mucosal surface of the upper respiratory passages.

HISTOGENESIS OF SALIVARY GLAND TUMORS

The inductive influences for salivary gland neoplasms are not well understood. Epithelial tumors may arise from any cell type of the salivary gland-excretory duct system, and the classification of these tumors is invariably tied to various histogenetic theories. For the purposes of this text, it is more fruitful to consider the relationship of the various tumors to their corresponding precursor cell types as taxonomic rather than histogenetic (Table 1-1).

Table 1-1. *World Health Organization histologic classification of salivary gland tumors (1992)*

1 Adenomas
    1.1 Pleomorphic adenoma
    1.2 Myoepithelioma (myoepithelial adenoma)
    1.3 Basal cell adenoma
    1.4 Warthin's tumor (adenolymphoma)
    1.5 Oncocytoma (oncocytic adenoma)
    1.6 Canalicular adenoma
    1.7 Sebaceous adenoma
    1.8 Ductal papilloma
        1.8.1 Inverted ductal papilloma
        1.8.2 Intraductal papilloma
        1.8.3 Sialadenoma papilliferum
    1.9 Cystadenoma
        1.9.1 Papillary cystadenoma
        1.9.2 Mucinous cystadenoma
2 Carcinomas
    2.1 Acinic cell carcinoma
    2.2 Mucoepidermoid carcinoma
    2.3 Adenoid cystic carcinoma
    2.4 Polymorphous low-grade adenocarcinoma (terminal duct adenocarcinoma)
    2.5 Epithelial-myoepithelial carcinoma
    2.6 Basal cell adenocarcinoma
    2.7 Sebaceous carcinoma
    2.8 Papillary cystadenocarcinoma
    2.9 Mucinous adenocarcinoma
    2.10 Oncocytic carcinoma
    2.11 Salivary duct carcinoma
    2.12 Adenocarcinoma
    2.13 Malignant myoepithelioma (myoepithelial carcinoma)
    2.14 Squamous cell carcinoma
    2.15 Small-cell carcinoma
    2.16 Undifferentiated carcinoma
    2.17 Other carcinomas
3 Nonepithelial tumors
4 Malignant lymphomas
5 Secondary tumors
6 Unclassified tumors
7 Tumorlike lesions
    7.1 Sialadenosis
    7.2 Oncocytosis
    7.3 Necrotizing sialometaplasia (salivary gland infarction)
    7.4 Benign lymphoepithelial lesion
    7.5 Salivary gland cysts
    7.6 Chronic sclerosing sialadenitis of submandibular gland (Küttner tumor)
    7.7 Cystic lymphoid hyperplasia in patients with acquired immunodeficiency syndrome

HISTOLOGY OF BENIGN TUMORS

Pleomorphic Adenoma

Pleomorphic adenoma (benign mixed tumor) is the most common salivary gland tumor. Although the histologic appearance of pleomorphic adenoma is quite variable, a constant feature is the presence of both epithelial and stromal components. The seemingly unlimited histologic variability results from the interplay of its two constituent cells: myoepithelial and ductal epithelial. The tumors are well circumscribed and are surrounded by a pseudocapsule of fibrous tissue. The epithelial elements demonstrate tubular and cordlike arrangements. The cells are round and contain a moderate amount of cytoplasm. Squamous metaplasia is frequently seen, and focal cytologic atypia is not uncommon. Mitoses are rare, and when increased in number, they signify possible malignant transformation. Although infarction may occur, tumor necrosis should alert the pathologist to the possibility of malignant transformation or prior damage from a fine-needle biopsy.

The stromal or "mesenchymal" component can be quite variable and is attributable to the myoepithelial cells. Most tumors show areas of chondroid (cartilaginous) differentiation. Osseous metaplasia is not uncommon. For the most part, the stroma is relatively hypocellular and composed of pale blue to slightly eosinophilic tissue containing occasional angulated cells and occasional ductlike or epithelial structures. Generally, the myoepithelial elements dominate. When epithelial elements comprise 10% or less of an apparent pleomorphic adenoma, it qualifies as a myoepithelioma.

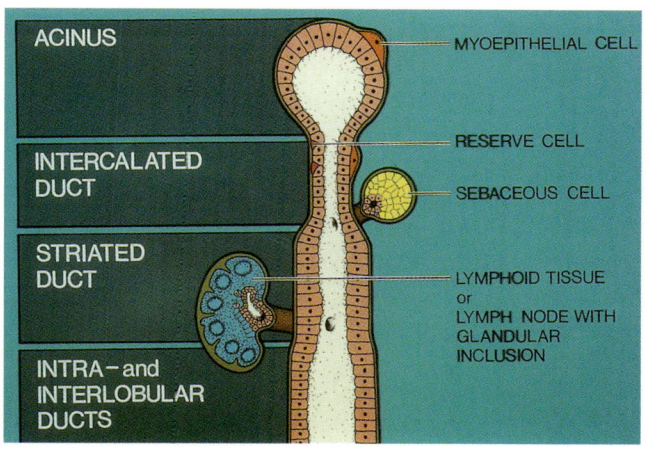

FIG. 1-1. Schematic of the salivary duct unit, from which its tumors originate.

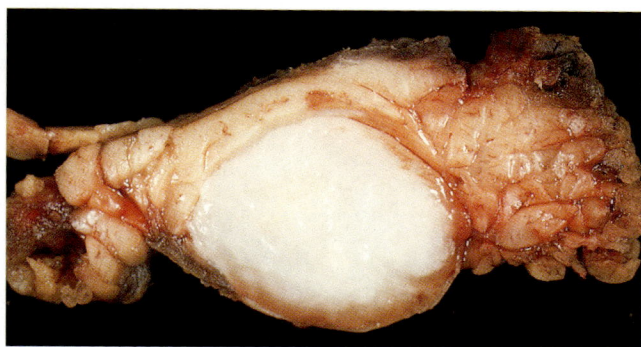

FIG. 1-2. Pleomorphic adenoma of parotid gland with glistening "chondroid" cut surface.

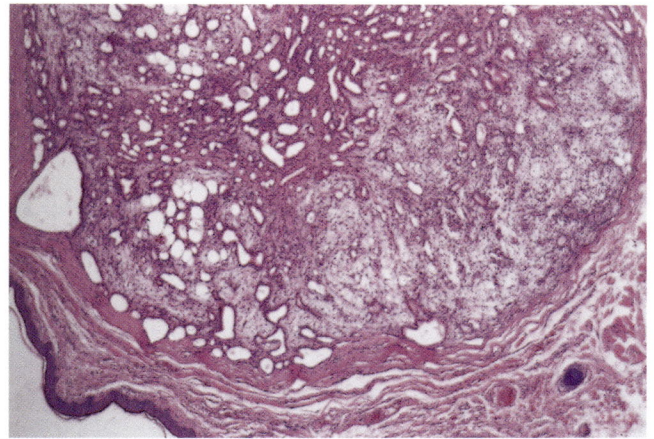

FIG. 1-3. Pleomorphic adenoma of nasal septum.

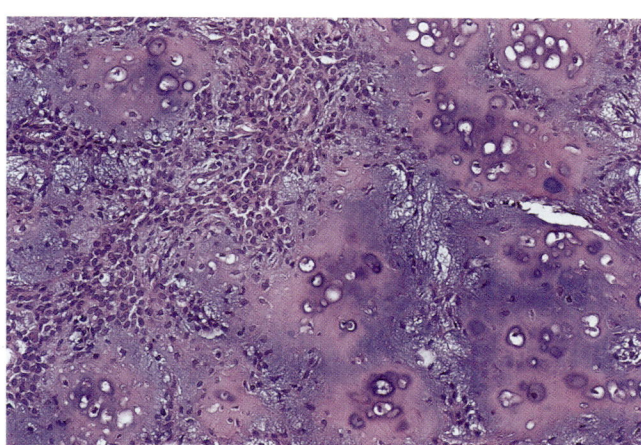

FIG. 1-4. Cartilaginous stroma in a pleomorphic adenoma.

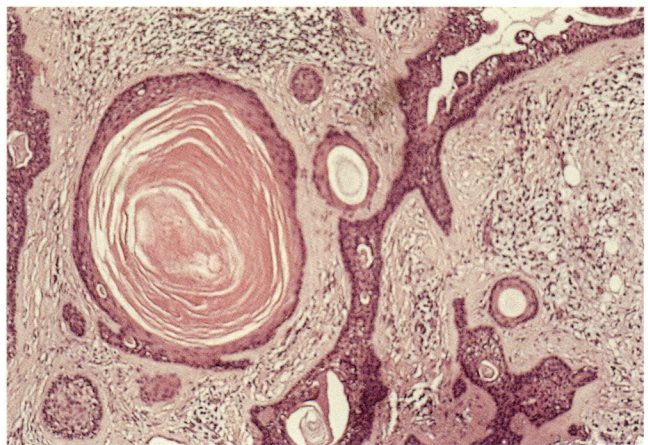

FIG. 1-5. Squamous metaplasia in a pleomorphic adenoma.

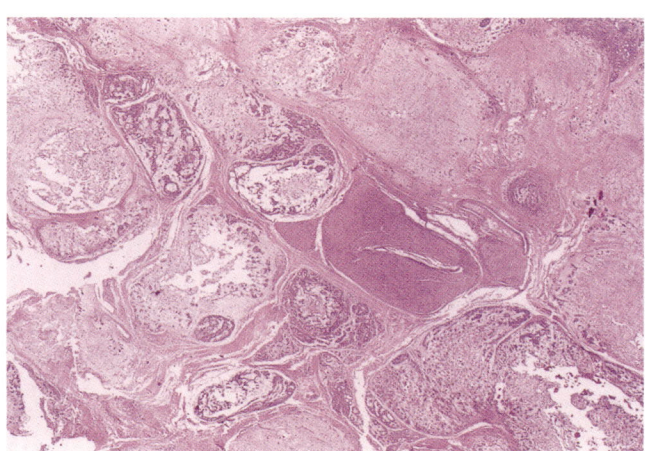

FIG. 1-6. Recurrent pleomorphic adenoma surrounding facial nerve.

Warthin's Tumor

Warthin's tumor (adenolymphoma, cystadenoma lymphomatosum) is the second most common tumor of the parotid gland and occurs almost exclusively there. Occasional cases are seen in the submandibular gland.

The tumor is thought to arise from salivary gland inclusions within lymph nodes. The epithelial component consists of papillary fronds, which demonstrate two layers of oncocytic epithelial cells. These are the distinguishing cells of Warthin's tumor and are the salivary homologue of Hürthle cells. These cells have small nuclei that frequently exhibit palisading away from the basement membrane. The cytoplasm of the epithelial cell stains a deep pink color on routine preparations and shows prominent granularity by virtue of a superabundance of mitochondria. Occasionally, the epithelium will undergo squamous metaplasia. Although this should present no diagnostic dilemma during examination of histologic sections, a mistaken diagnosis of squamous carcinoma might be made on evaluation of fine-needle aspiration biopsy material. Mucous cell hypertrophy may at times be seen, and when present with squamous metaplasia, it can be mistaken for mucoepidermoid carcinoma.

In addition to the epithelial component, there is an abundance of normal lymphoid tissue. Occasional germinal centers will be seen. This lymphoid tissue forms the "core" of the papillary structures. Both lymphoid and oncocytic epithelial elements must be present for a diagnosis of Warthin's tumor to be made.

The tumor frequently has a prominent cystic component. Cystic fluid is usually grayish brown and will contain histiocytes and rare epithelial fragments. The tumor is more often bilateral than other types, and it is also more frequently associated with synchronous or metachronous multicentricity within the same gland.

Monomorphic Adenomas

Basal Cell Adenoma

Basal cell adenomas are relatively uncommon, accounting for 2% of all salivary gland tumors. They occur almost exclusively in the major glands, with the parotid gland being the most frequently affected site. The tumors are encapsulated, well-circumscribed masses with occasional cystic change. They are composed of a predominance of epithelial cells, which resemble the basal or "reserve" cells of the intercalated duct. The tumors manifest a variety of growth patterns, including solid, tubular, trabecular, and membranous. Combinations of growth patterns are common.

The membranous pattern is so named because of the excessive replication of basal lamina or "basement membrane-like" material that is found between nests and cords of epithelial cells. This particular subtype bears great similarity to certain dermal appendage tumors, particularly eccrine spiradenoma and dermal cylindroma, hence the term dermal analogue tumor. The membranous pattern has been associated with the concurrent development of these skin tumors, which is known as the salivary gland-skin tumor syndrome. Dermal analogue tumors are more likely to be multicentric and recur more frequently than other types. Although malignant degeneration is rare, it is seen more frequently with the membranous subtype.

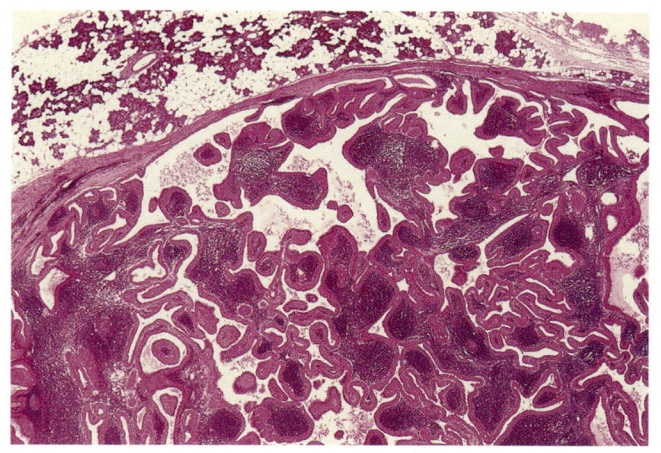
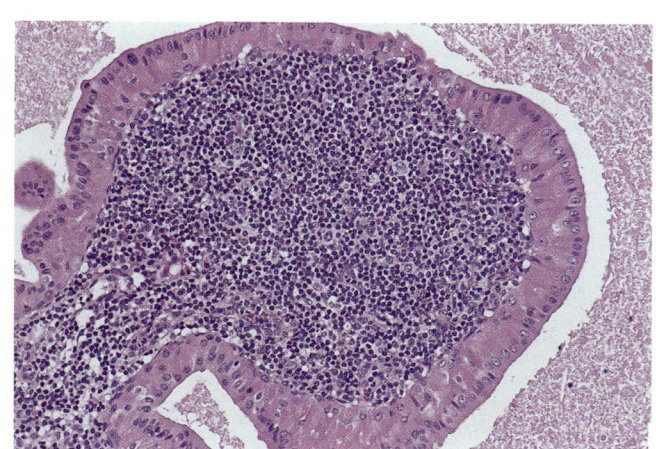
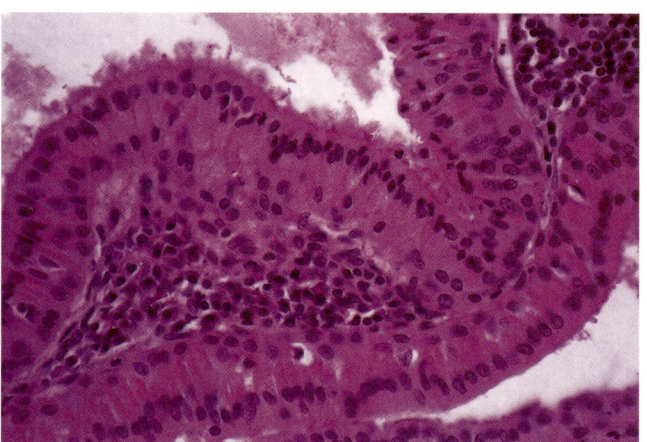

FIG. 1-7. A–C: Warthin's tumor, with its bicellular composition of oncocytes and lymphoid cells.

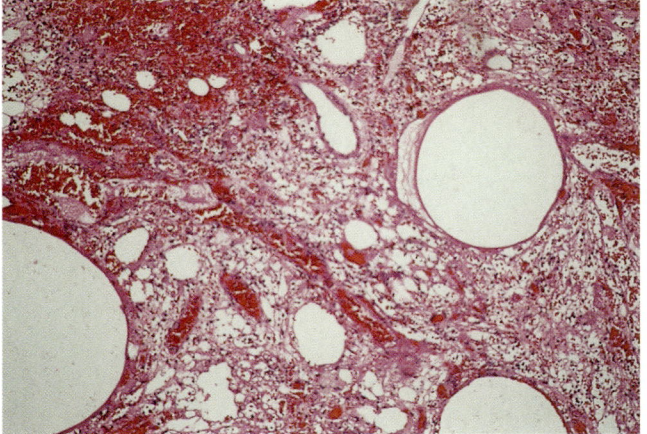

FIG. 1-8. Lipidic necrosis of Warthin's tumor after fine-needle aspiration.

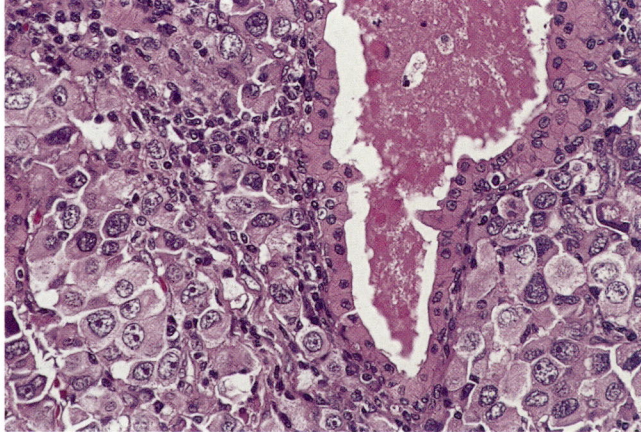

FIG. 1-9. High-grade carcinoma arising in Warthin's tumor.

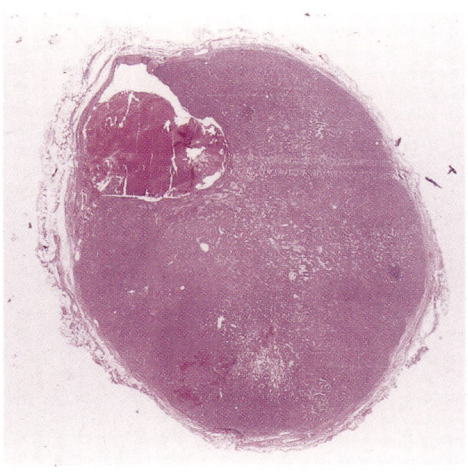

FIG. 1-10. Monomorphic adenoma. Note the absence of stromal changes in an epithelial tumor.

Oncocytoma

Oncocytomas are histologically similar to Warthin's tumors, except that no lymphoid tissue is present. The oncocytic cells may be arranged in a villous pattern of growth but are more commonly arranged in small, tightly packed clusters. The tumors are well circumscribed and occur almost exclusively in the major salivary glands, especially the parotid. Mitoses are not common, and their presence should alert the pathologist to the risk of malignant transformation, an event that occurs only rarely.

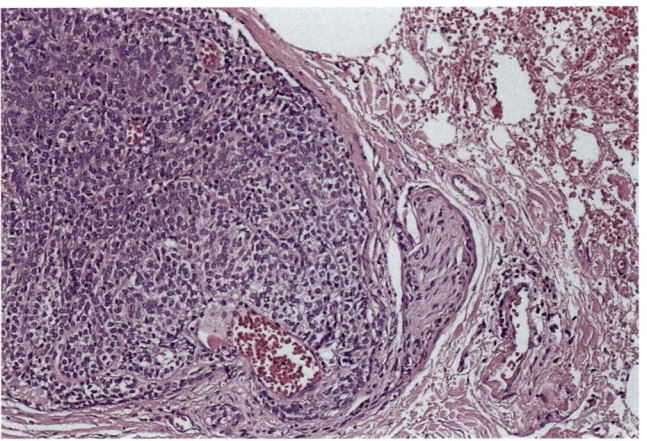

FIG. 1-11. Dermal analogue tumor approaching small nerve.

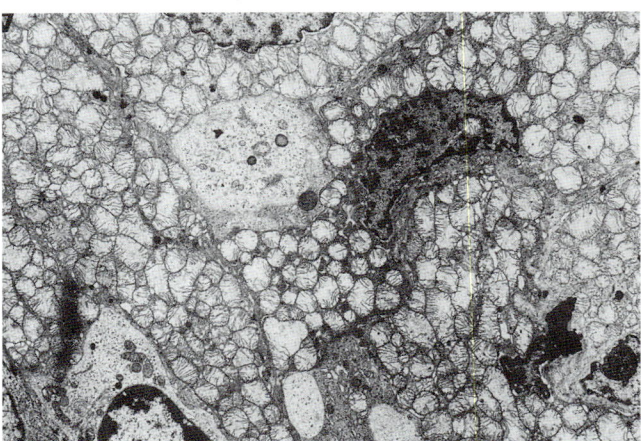

FIG. 1-12. Epithelial cells filled with mitochondria, the defining constituents of oncocytes.

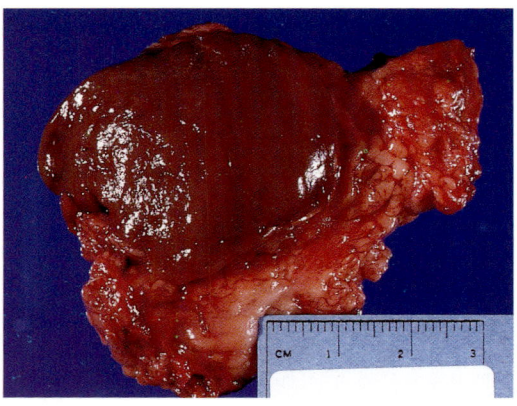

FIG. 1-13. Oncocytoma of parotid gland with typical circumscription and color.

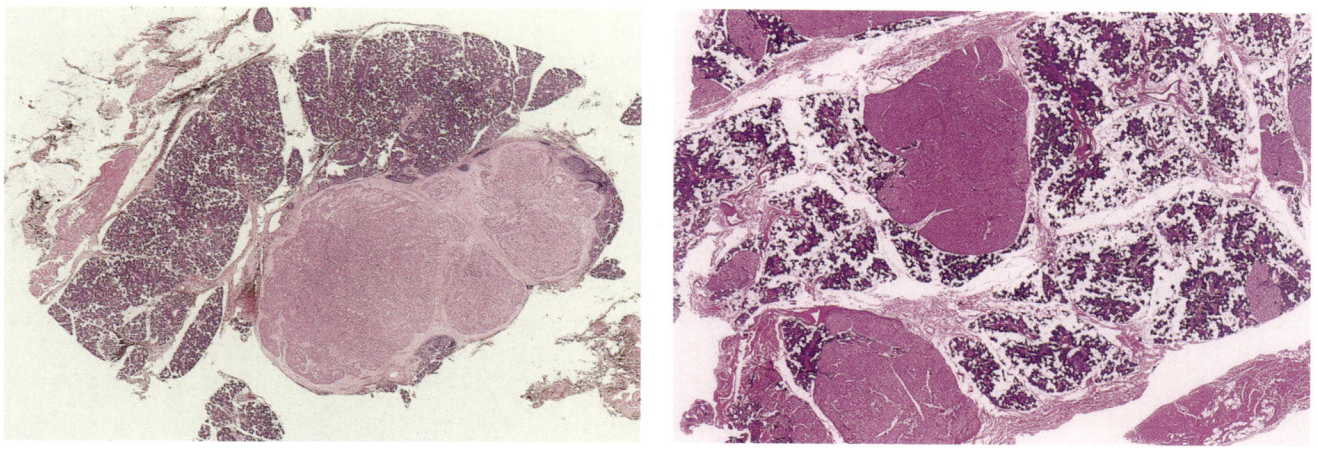

FIG. 1-14. A,B: Oncocytoma of parotid gland in **A**. Compare with oncocytosis in **B**.

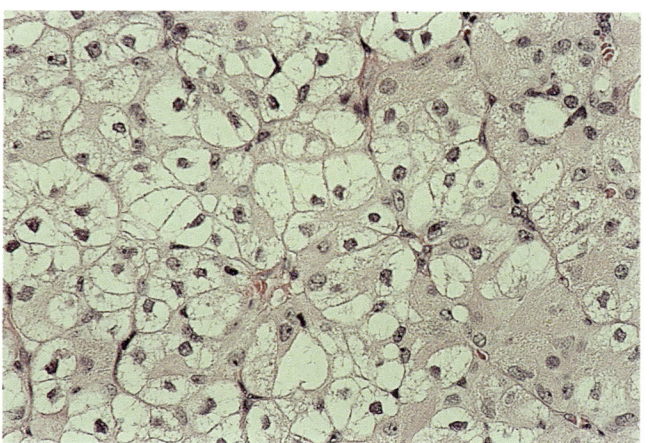

FIG. 1-15. Clear cell change in oncocytic cells of an oncocytoma.

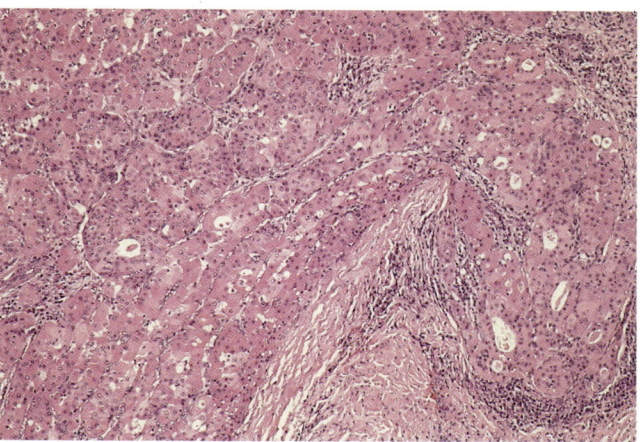

FIG. 1-16. Aggressive oncocytoma of parotid gland showing nodular invasion of stroma.

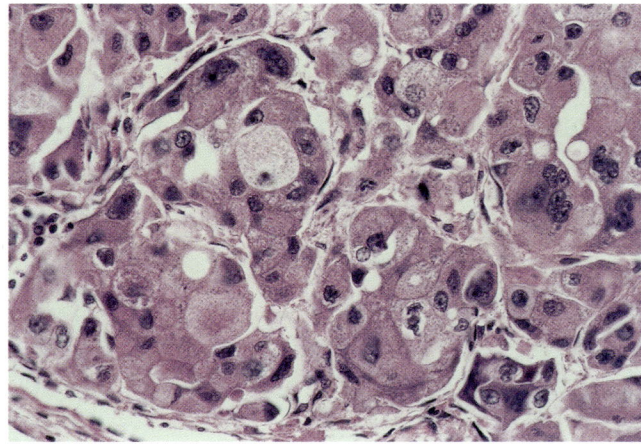

FIG. 1-17. Oncocytic carcinoma.

Canalicular Adenoma

Canalicular adenoma is a tumor histogenically related to basal cell adenoma, but with distinct morphologic and clinical characteristics. These tumors tend to occur in the minor salivary glands, especially those of the upper lip, where they present as bluish masses. The tumors are not encapsulated, and multicentric involvement within the gland is typical and should not be confused with an invasive process.

The tumor is composed of medium-sized basal cells that occasionally form trabeculae and rests with peripheral palisading of nuclei. The tumor secretes copious quantities of mucuslike material into the intercellular stroma, which causes cystic change resembling the pattern of growth seen in adenoid cystic carcinoma. In this tumor, however, residual stromal elements are seen within the cystlike spaces; these are not found in adenoid cystic carcinoma. The presence of capillaries and small blood vessels within the cystic areas is a very helpful diagnostic feature.

Inverted Ductal Papilloma

These lesions are histologically very similar to the inverted squamous papilloma of the sinonasal tract, and distinguishing the two may be difficult. Features that may be helpful include location of the lesion within a bed of salivary gland tissue, presence of columnar or mucous cells on the luminal surface, and presence of terminal duct elements.

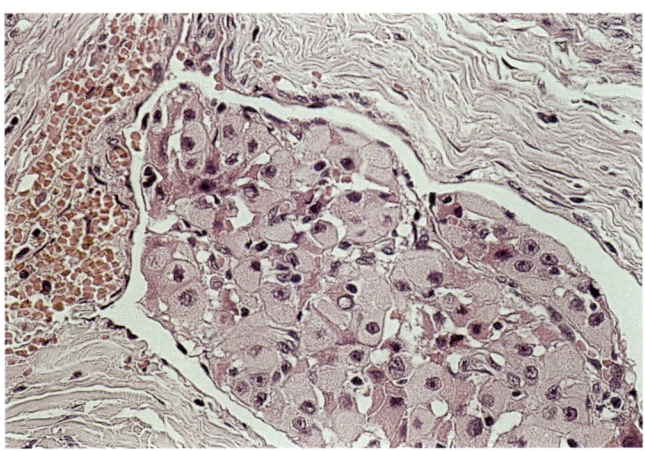

FIG. 1-18. Oncocytic carcinoma in vein.

A

B

C

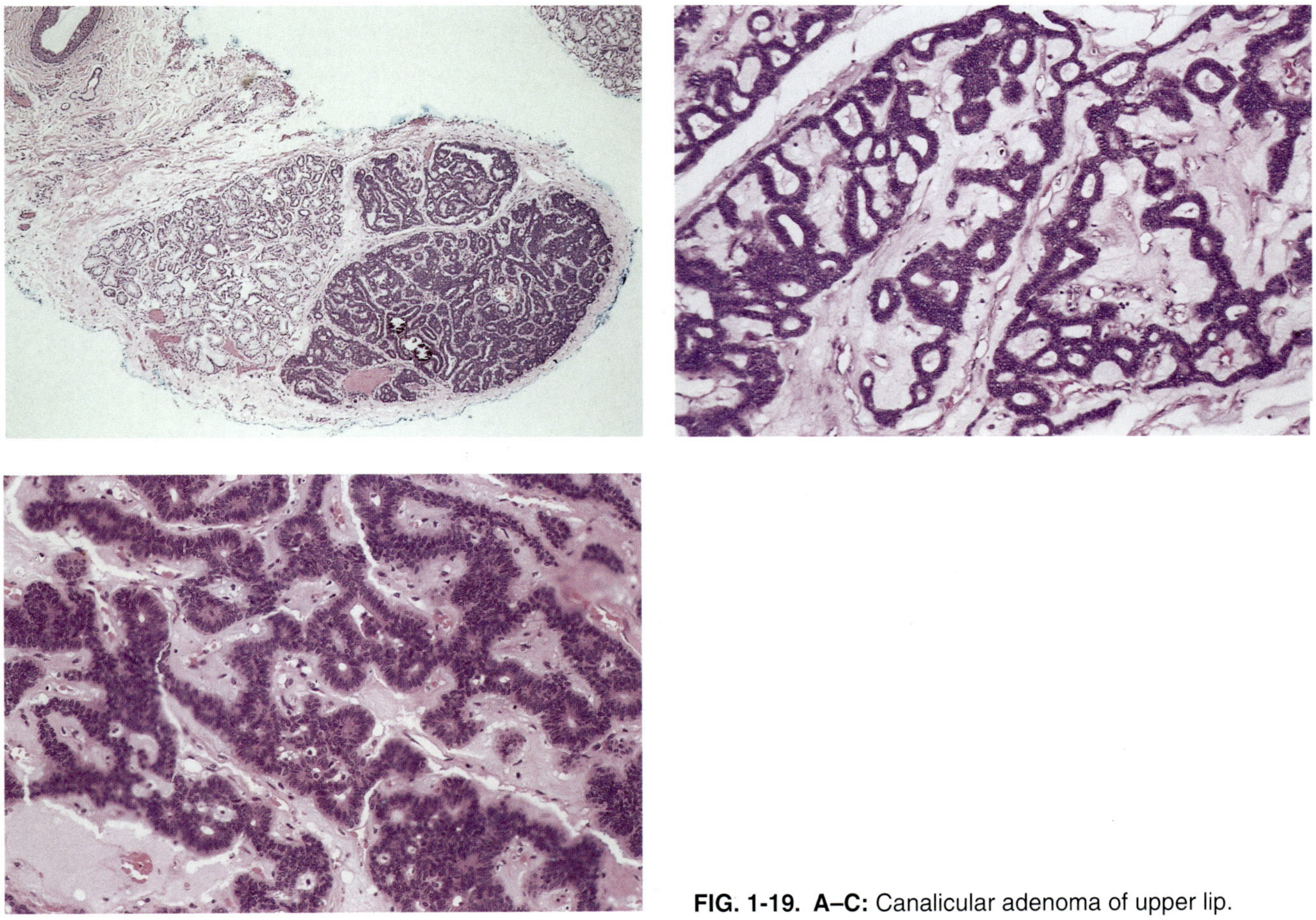

FIG. 1-19. A–C: Canalicular adenoma of upper lip.

Myoepithelioma

Myoepithelioma can be viewed as a monomorphic presentation of a pleomorphic adenoma exhibiting only myoepithelial cells. It is a rare tumor that accounts for fewer than 1% of pleomorphic adenomas. The diagnosis is difficult to make on light microscopy. Several cell types are described: plasmacytoid, clear, epitheloid, and spindled. The definitive diagnosis rests on electron microscopic and immunohistochemical confirmation of the myoepithelium.

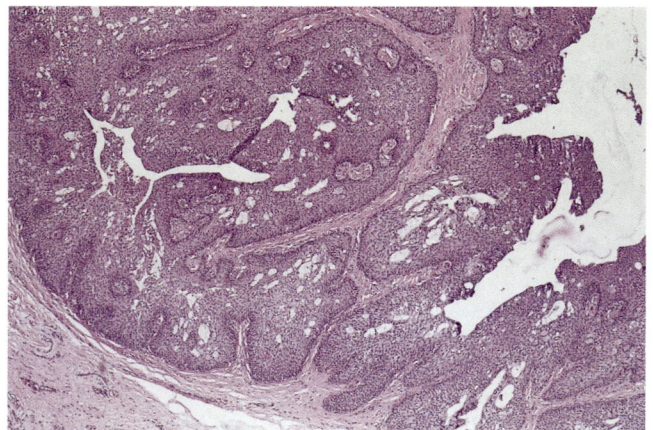 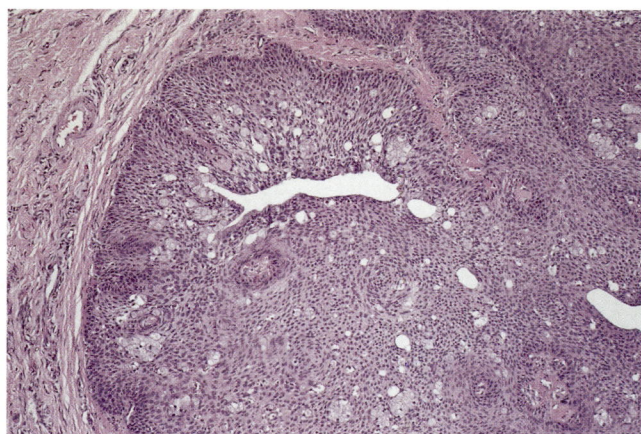

FIG. 1-20. A,B: Inverted ductal papilloma of the oral cavity. Except for a resemblance to schneiderian papillomas, there is no other relationship. The lesions are benign.

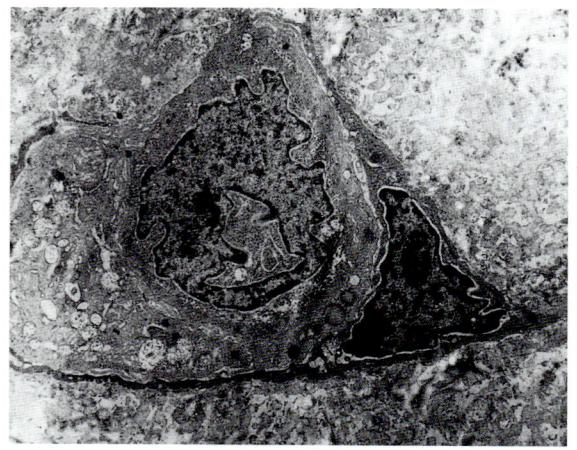 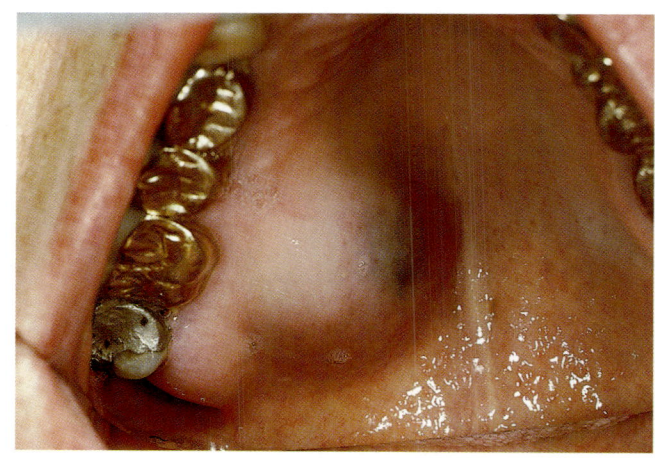

FIG. 1-21. Electron-optic appearance of a myoepithelial cell.

FIG. 1-22. Myoepithelioma of oral cavity.

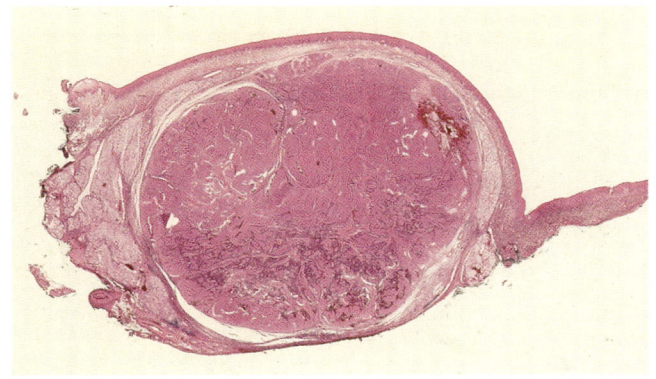

FIG. 1-23. Oral myoepithelioma.

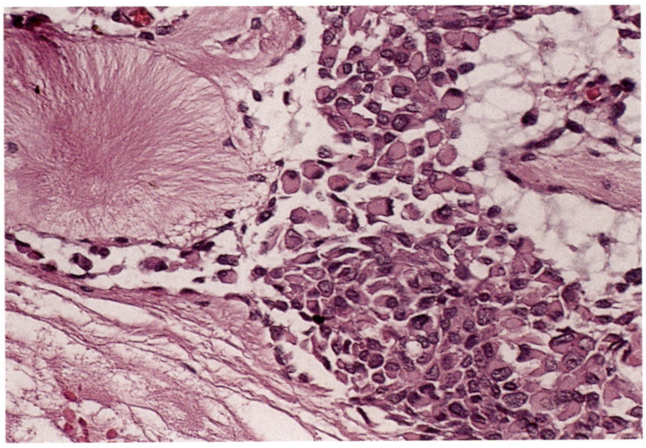

FIG. 1-24. A–C: Myoepithelioma with pathognomonic extracellular eosinophilic crystalloids.

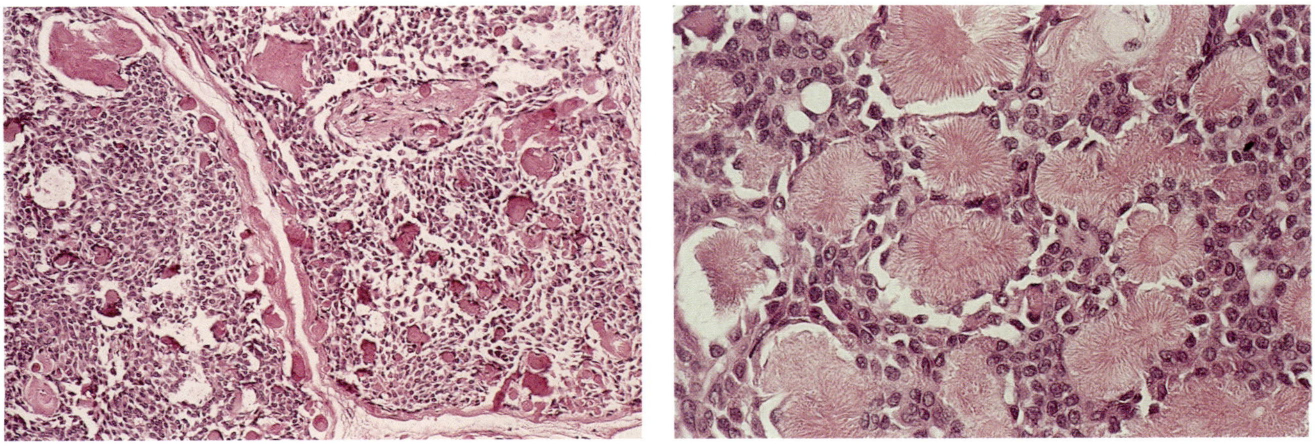

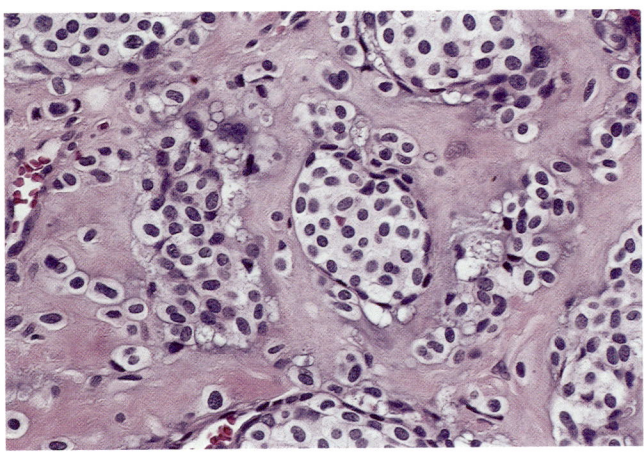

FIG. 1-25. Clear cell myoepithelioma.

Dermal Analogue Tumor Monomorphic Adenoma

This designation is used to describe monomorphic adenomas that have a resemblance to dermal appendage tumors. They are benign and quite rare. Multifocal origin may account for recurrences. Malignant transformation is the highest of any of the monomorphic adenomas.

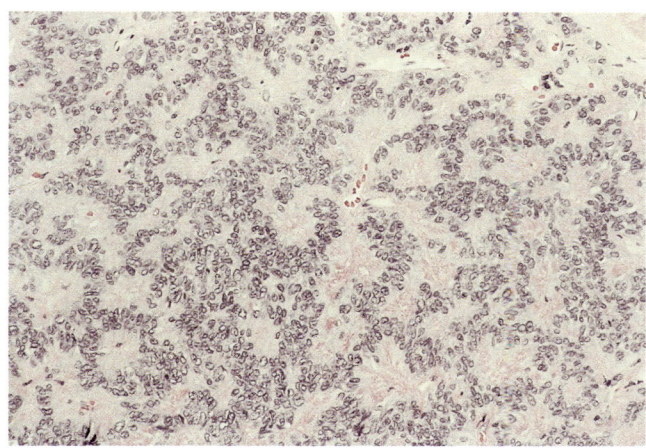

FIG. 1-26. Myoepithelioma after external radiation. Note radioresistant persistence.

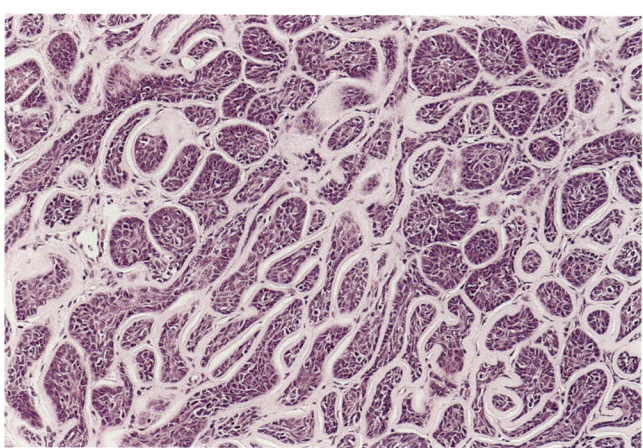

FIG. 1-27. Dermal analogue monomorphic adenoma of parotid gland.

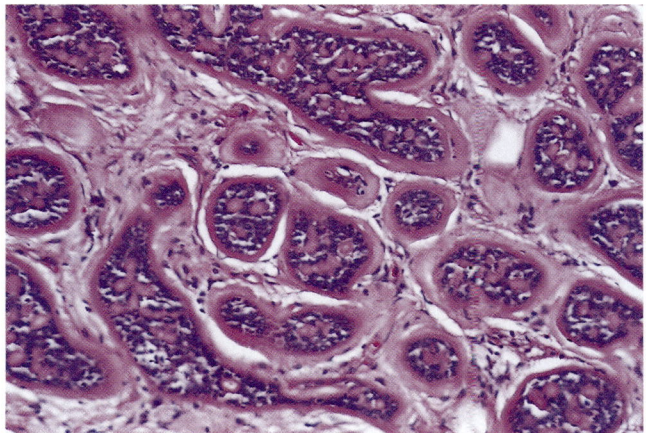

FIG. 1-28. Dermal analogue monomorphic adenoma of parotid gland. Note the thickened basement membrane material around the epithelial islands.

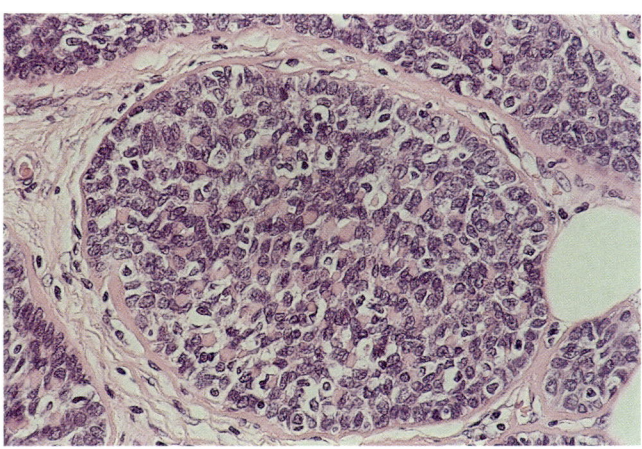

FIG. 1-29. Dermal analogue tumor with hyalinized basement membrane.

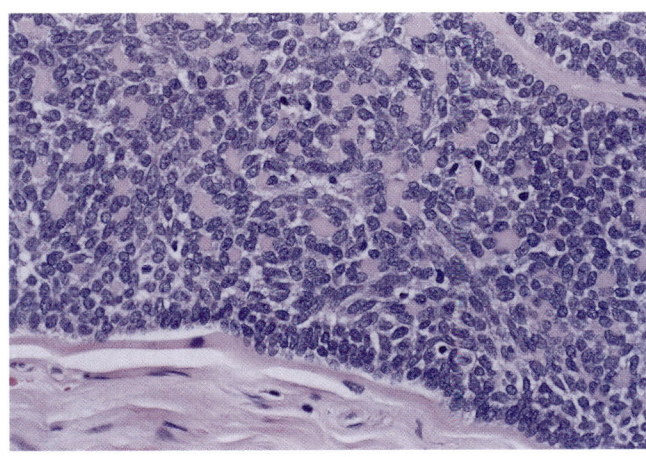

FIG. 1-30. Dermal analogue tumor with characteristic eosinophilic extracellular "droplets."

Sialoblastoma

Sialoblastoma (embryoma) is clinically manifested in neonates as a unilateral parotid mass. It arises in the fetus as a result of failure of the modulating interaction between embryonic ducts and primitive mesenchyme. This tumor is rare, and a malignant counterpart is even more so.

Sebaceous Tumors

Extracutaneous sebaceous glands are a normal finding in the anterior oral cavity, most often in the labial-buccal area, where they are given the eponymous designation of Fordyce's granules. In other salivary sites, they may be normal or metaplastic, especially in chronic inflammatory conditions.

Tumor-forming sebaceous lesions in salivary glands are the rarely occurring sebaceous adenoma and the more frequent sebaceous lymphadenoma. Sebaceous carcinomas found in the parotid or submandibular glands are more likely to be metastatic than primary.

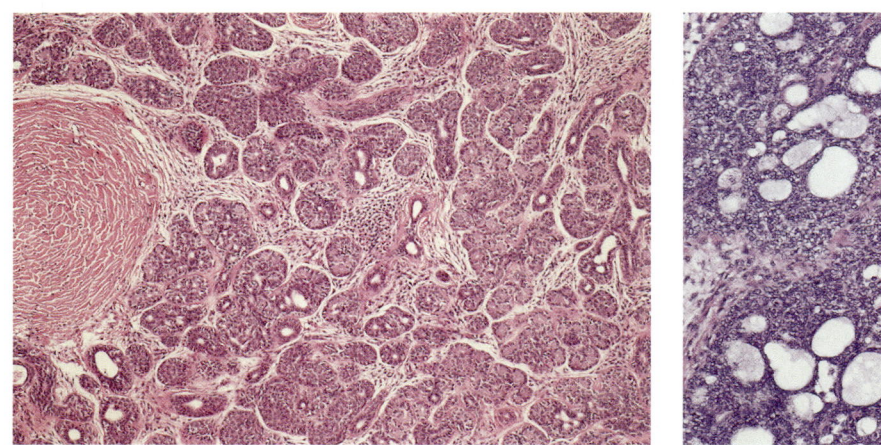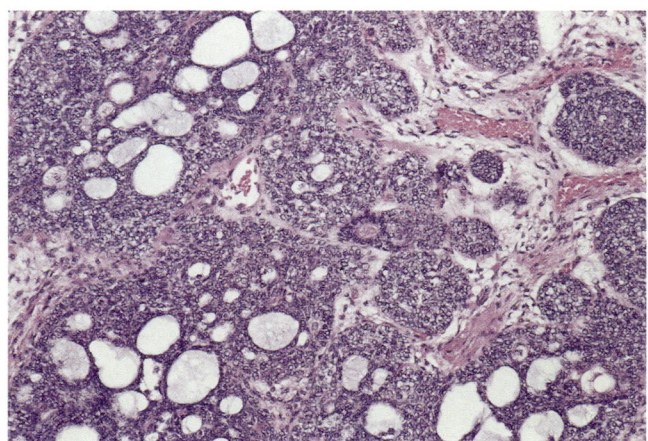

FIG. 1-31. A,B: Sialoblastoma (embryoma of neonatal parotid gland).

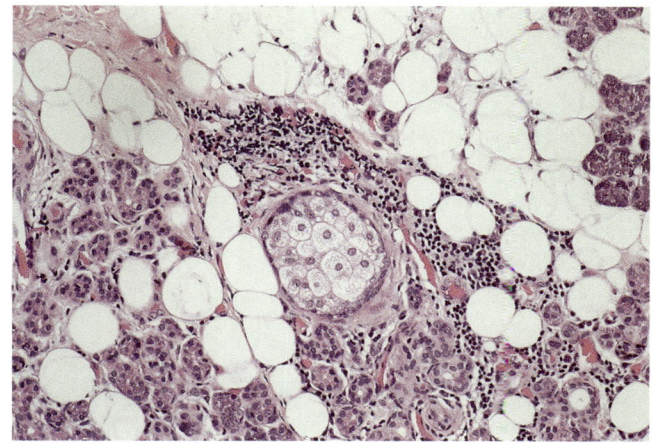

FIG. 1-32. Sebaceous focus in normal (child's) parotid gland.

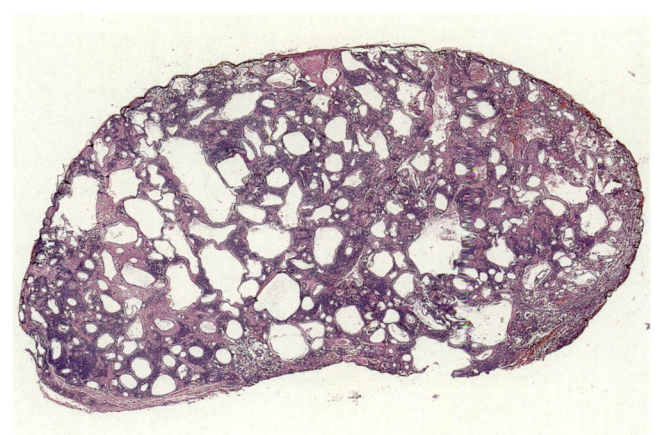
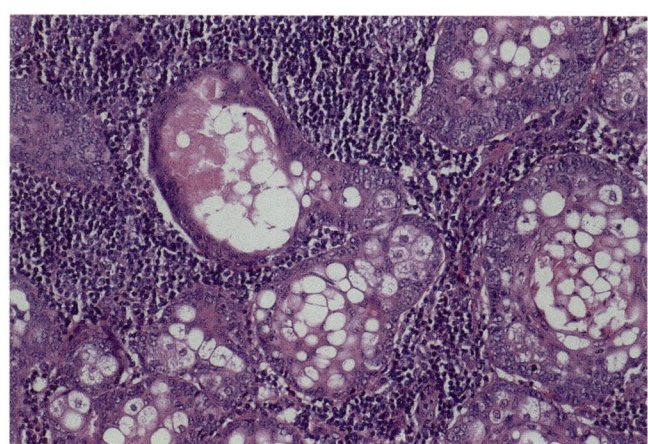

FIG. 1-33. A,B: Sebaceous lymphadenoma.

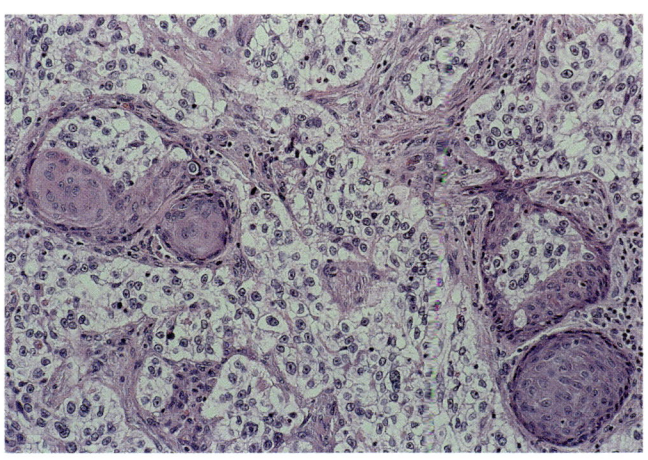

FIG. 1-34. Sebaceous carcinoma, apparently primary in the parotid gland.

HISTOLOGY OF MALIGNANT TUMORS

General Remarks

The morphologic varieties of malignant salivary gland tumors are numerous. Although cytologic characteristics are the key to the subclassification of tumors, architectural features generally provide a more reliable clue to clinical behavior. Hence, the behavior of a cytologically benign but diffusely infiltrating lesion will be more aggressive than that of a cytologically atypical but well-circumscribed tumor. This is probably more a consequence of successful extirpation than of true tumor biology, as diffusely infiltrating lesions are always more difficult to remove. Clinical stage is a better prognostic indicator than histomorphology.

Mucoepidermoid Carcinoma

Mucoepidermoid carcinoma was originally named for the two obvious cell types found in this tumor, mucous and epidermoid (squamouslike), but the intermediate cell is the linear progenitor of both. This is the most common malignant salivary gland tumor at any salivary site. Its clinical behavior is related to both stage and degree of differentiation. Well-differentiated tumors tend to present as localized, well-circumscribed masses, whereas poorly differentiated tumors tend to infiltrate and metastasize early. However, grade is less important than clinical stage as an indicator of prognosis.

Mucoepidermoid carcinomas are frequently cystic and may be associated with a prominent lymphocytic component. Differentiation is clearly tied to the quantity and character of the epidermoid component. Differentiation from squamous cell carcinoma in all cases rests on the identification of mucous cells, which decrease progressively with progressively poorer differentiation of a tumor. It should be appreciated that cornified squamous cells are never, or at best very rarely, seen. If they are present, the tumor is more likely a conventional squamous cell carcinoma.

Well-differentiated mucoepidermoid carcinoma demonstrates a preponderance of mucous cells with a relatively small epidermoid component. The epidermoid component comprises two cell types: a more mature form, which is similar to squamous epithelium, and a relatively immature cell, the "intermediate" cell. This cell contains a somewhat larger nucleus than the epidermoid cell and a moderate amount of pale pink-staining cytoplasm. It has a distinct tendency to undergo "clear cell" change, which is most likely an artifact of fixation.

The epidermoid component may be sparse but is usually easily identified, and it is rarely atypical. A histologically malignant epidermoid component is better considered a less well-differentiated tumor. Extravasated mucus is a common feature of well-differentiated tumors, sometimes forming the predominant component histologically and leading to sclerosis.

Moderately differentiated mucoepidermoid carcinoma shows more intermediate and fewer mucous cells. The "intermediate" epidermoid cell may predominate, and clear cells may make up a large component. Mucous cells are readily identifiable. Mitoses become more common and are seen in the epidermoid component.

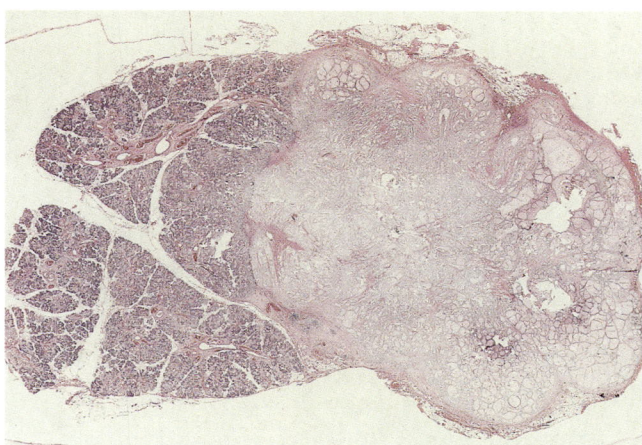

FIG. 1-35. Mucoepidermoid carcinoma of parotid gland.

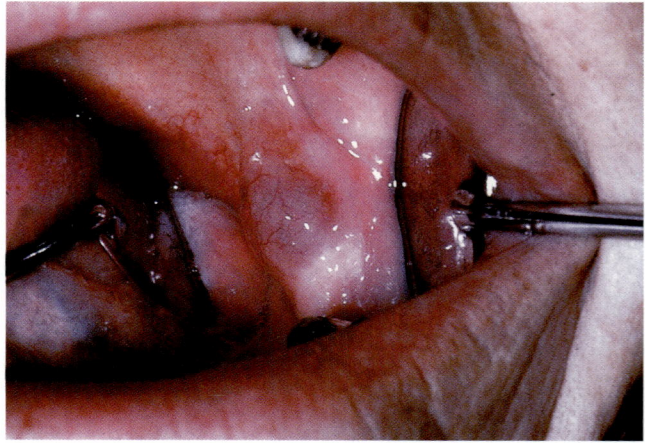

FIG. 1-36. Low-grade mucoepidermoid carcinoma of oral cavity.

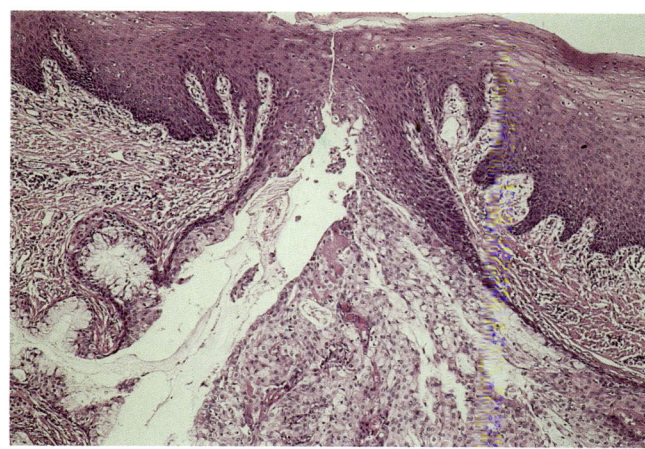

FIG. 1-37. Oral low-grade mucoepidermoid carcinoma. Note that the carcinoma is not a surface mucosal lesion.

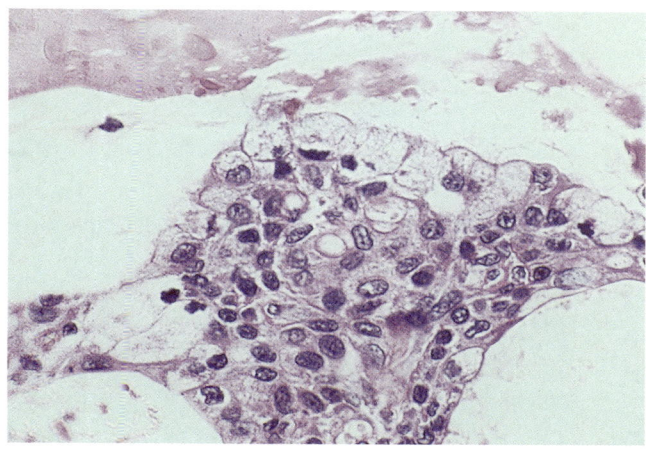

FIG. 1-38. Low-grade mucoepidermoid carcinoma. This papillary focus shows intermediate cells surrounded by mucous cells.

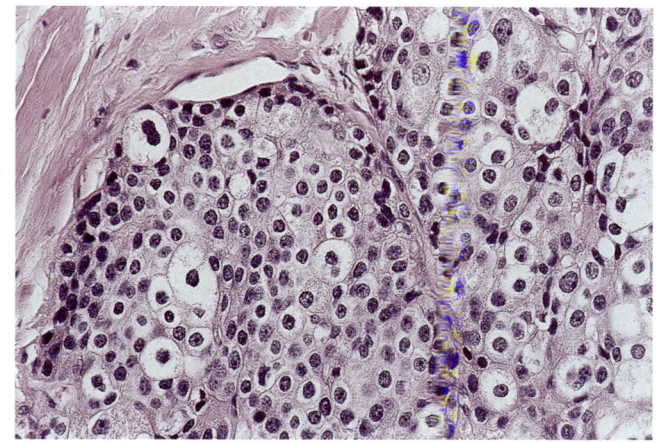

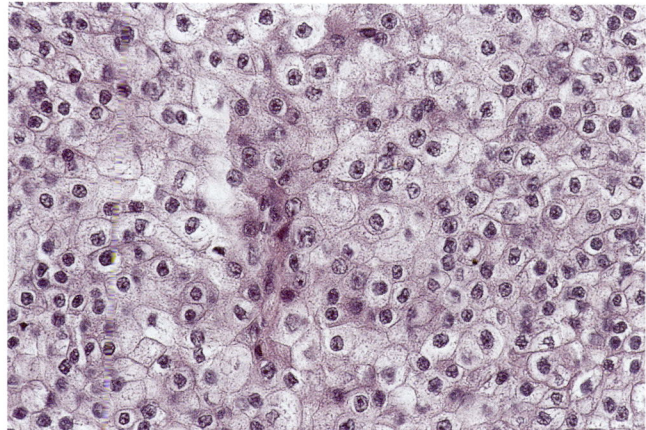

FIG. 1-39. A,B: Intermediate (grade 2) mucoepidermoid carcinoma with a cellular composition of intermediate cells.

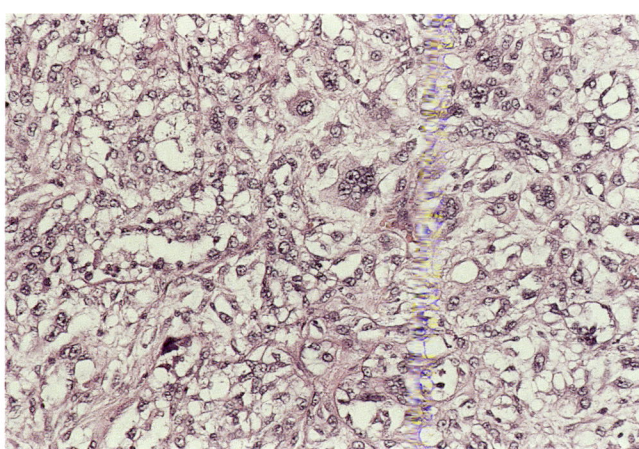

FIG. 1-40. High-grade (grade 3) mucoepidermoid carcinoma.

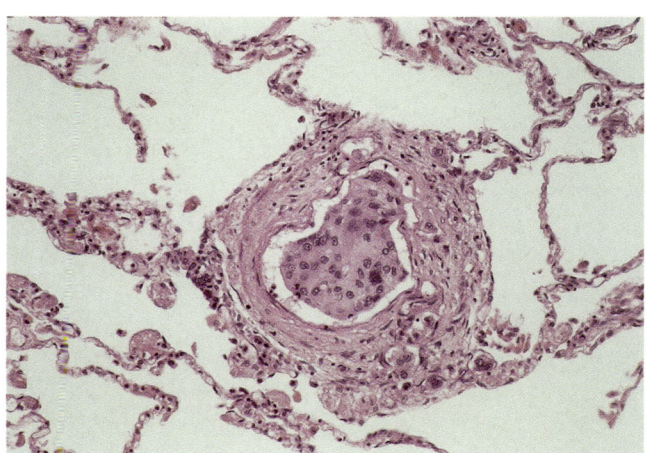

FIG. 1-41. Metastatic mucoepidermoid carcinoma in a pulmonary artery.

Poorly differentiated mucoepidermoid carcinoma can resemble a squamous cell carcinoma or a poorly differentiated adenocarcinoma, both cytologically as well as architecturally. Mucous cells are rare. Special stains for mucin are helpful and may be necessary to distinguish this tumor from primary (and importantly) metastatic squamous carcinoma. Mitoses are abundant and may be atypical.

Acinic Cell Adenocarcinoma

Acinic cell adenocarcinoma contains a variety of cell types and manifests multiple growth patterns. A rather consistent microscopic feature, however, is the presence of cells morphologically similar to the normal serous acinar cells. Of malignant tumors, it is third in frequency among adults and second among children.

The tumor is more likely to be found in the major salivary glands, especially the parotid, and usually presents as a well-circumscribed nodular mass. Origin in minor salivary glands is so infrequent that it should be questioned. The architectural cytologic features are variable and have been well elucidated by Abrams (Table 1-2). This tumor will only rarely contain a uniform cell type. There are no reliable histologic criteria to predict clinical outcome, and clinical staging is the most important single predictor of prognosis. The tumor is usually a low-grade carcinoma and can be expected to be less aggressive than other salivary carcinomas. There is a so-called "dedifferentiated" form that is high-grade and can be rapidly lethal.

Malignant Mixed Tumor

The term malignant mixed tumor can refer to a variety of histopathologic and clinical entities. It is important to separate the categories, as they respond differently to therapy and belong in different prognostic groups.

Table 1-2. *Acinic cell adenocarcinoma (after Abrams)*

Cell types	Growth patterns
Acinar	Solid
Intercalated ductlike	Microcystic
Vacuolated	Papillary-cystic
Clear	Follicular
Nonspecific ductlike	

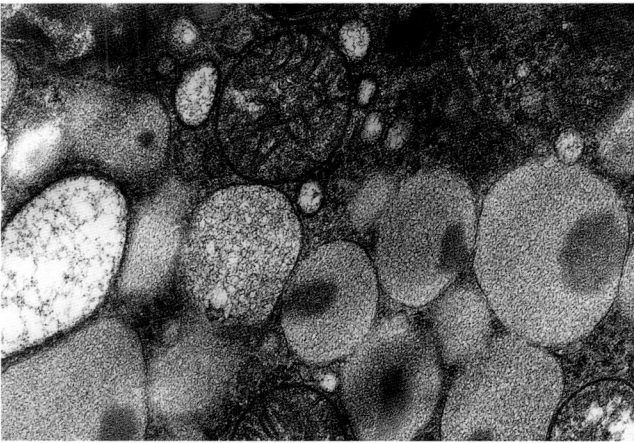

FIG. 1-42. Electron-optic appearance of an acinic cell carcinoma.

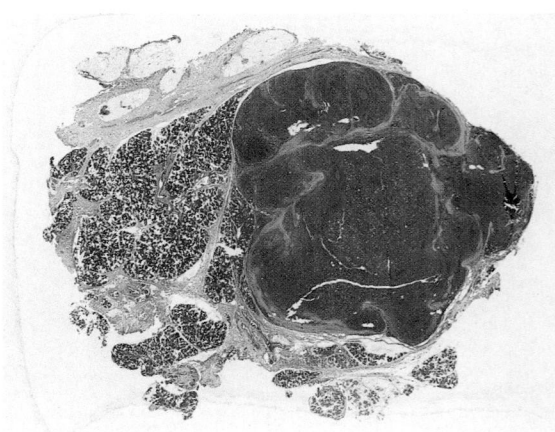

FIG. 1-43. Acinic cell carcinoma of parotid gland.

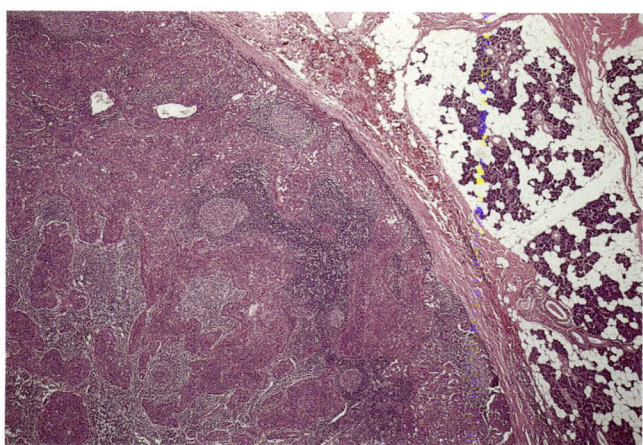

FIG. 1-44. Intranodal acinic cell carcinoma. The carcinoma arises from nodal inclusions of salivary tissue.

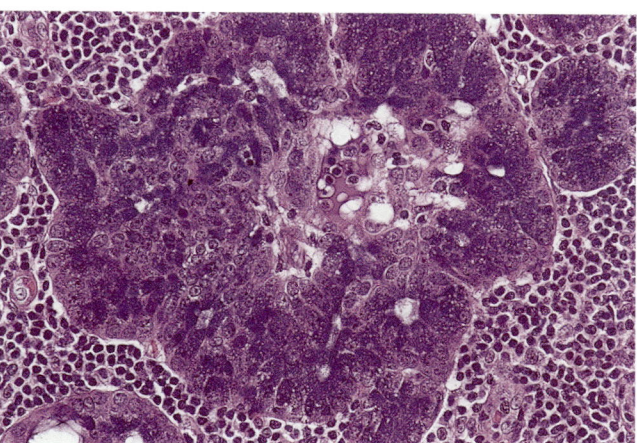

FIG. 1-45. So-called "blue-dot" acinic cell carcinoma. The intense basophilia is occasioned by secretory granules. The lymphoid cell accompaniment is often noted.

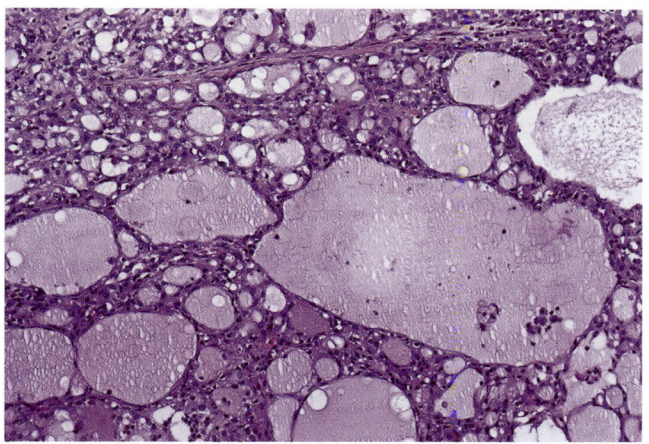

FIG. 1-46. Follicular pattern in an acinic cell carcinoma.

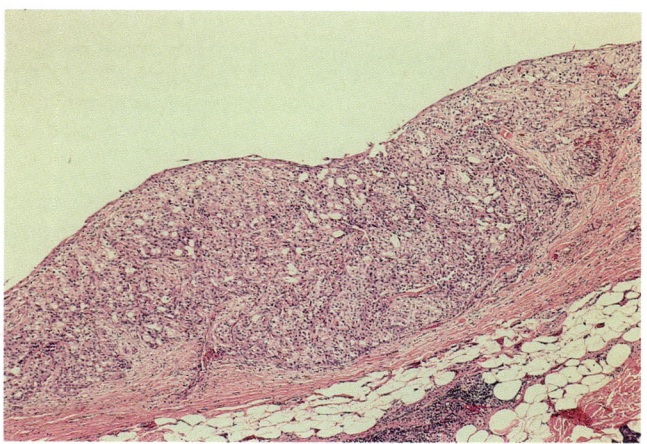

FIG. 1-47. Cystic acinic cell carcinoma.

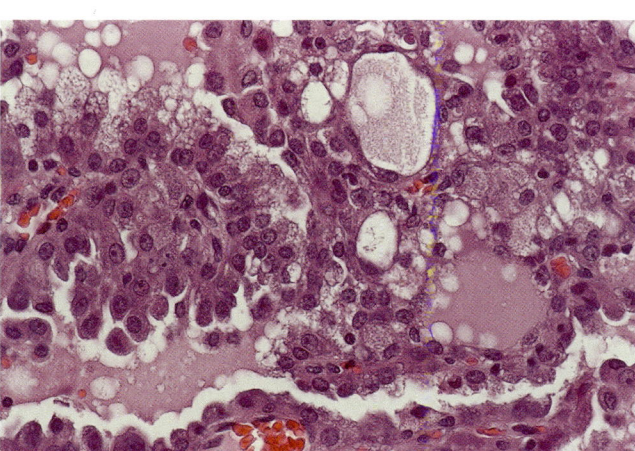

FIG. 1-48. Papillocystic acinic cell carcinoma.

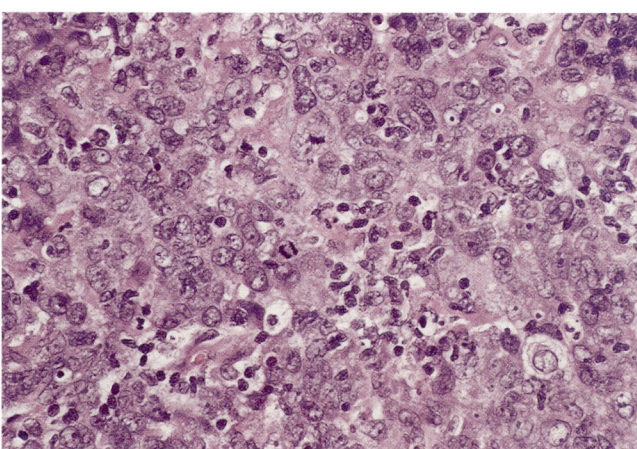

FIG. 1-49. High-grade (grade 3) acinic cell carcinoma of parotid gland. This undifferentiated carcinoma has a high rate of rapid mortality.

Benign Metastasizing Mixed Tumor

The appearance of this tumor is like that of pleomorphic adenoma, but it occurs as a metastatic lesion in patients with a history of previous benign mixed tumor. It is thought that metastasis develops as a result of tumor seeding of the vascular bed of the surgical field. It is exceedingly rare.

Carcinoma ex Pleomorphic Adenoma

In this most common form of "malignant mixed tumor," a ductal carcinoma arises from the ductal elements of a pleomorphic adenoma (Table 1-3). The carcinoma is usually invasive, but on occasion it may be confined to the maternal adenoma, a form of "carcinoma *in situ*." Carcinoma ex pleomorphic adenoma is the most common form of malignant mixed tumor. The risk for malignancy developing within a benign mixed tumor increases with time and is thought to be in the range of 5% to 7%.

Table 1-3. *Carcinoma ex pleomorphic adenoma*

Clinical and radiologic features	Pathologic features
Rapid growth in preexistent lesion of long duration	Elevated mitotic rate
Pain and nerve paralysis	Tissue infiltration, especially perineural invasion
Cystic degeneration (CT)	Necrosis
Microcalcifications (CT)	Microcalcifications
Regional lymph node enlargement	Lymph node or distant metastases
	Sclerosis with entrapment of epithelial elements

CT, computed tomography.

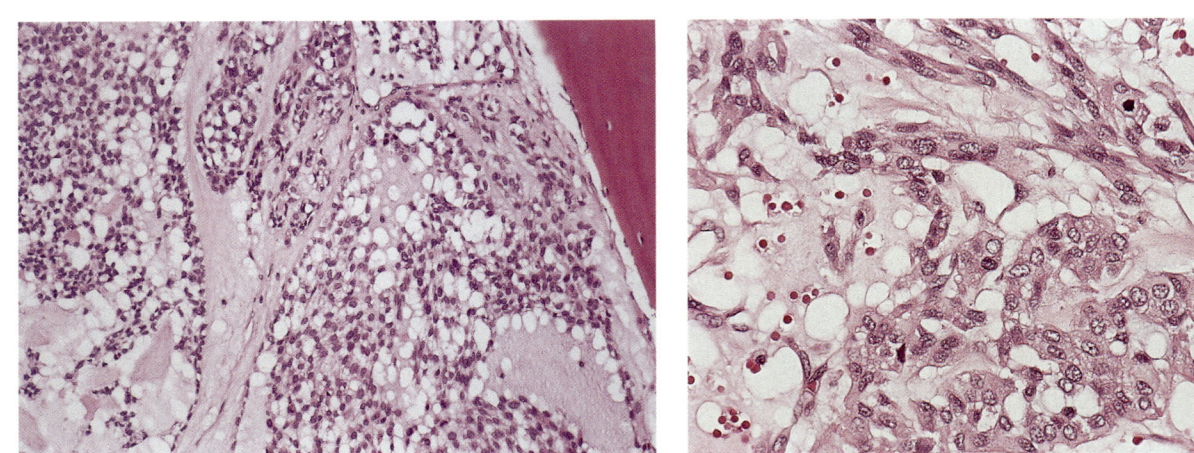

FIG. 1-50. A,B: One cytomorphologic form of so-called "benign metastasizing pleomorphic adenoma." A metastatic focus in bone is shown in A; the primary with myoepithelial features and mitoses appears in B.

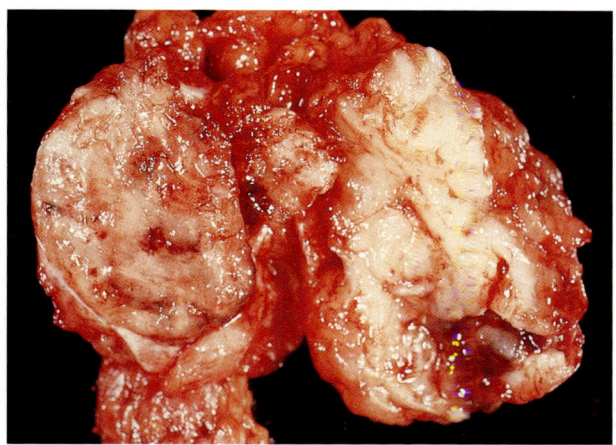

FIG. 1-51. Carcinoma ex pleomorphic adenoma of parotid gland manifesting cystic necrosis and nodular irregularity.

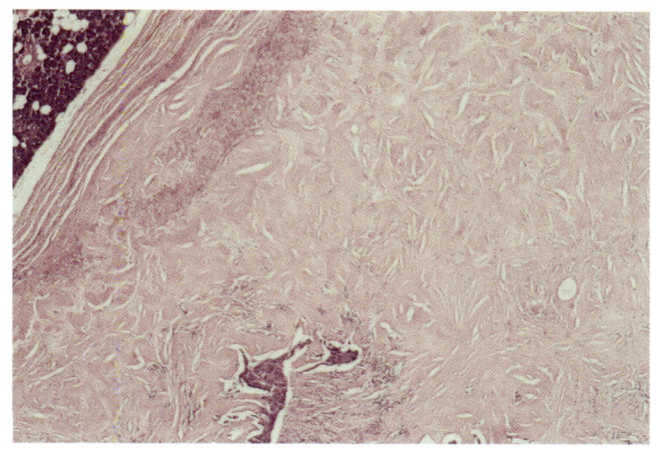

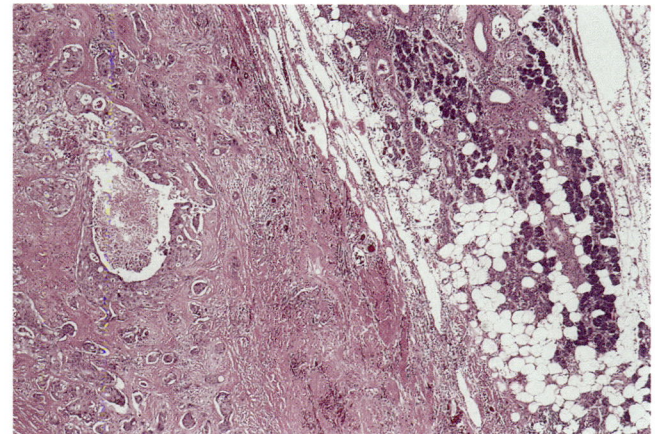

FIG. 1-52. A,B: Carcinoma ex pleomorphic adenoma. Dense hyalinization entraps scant malignant ducts.

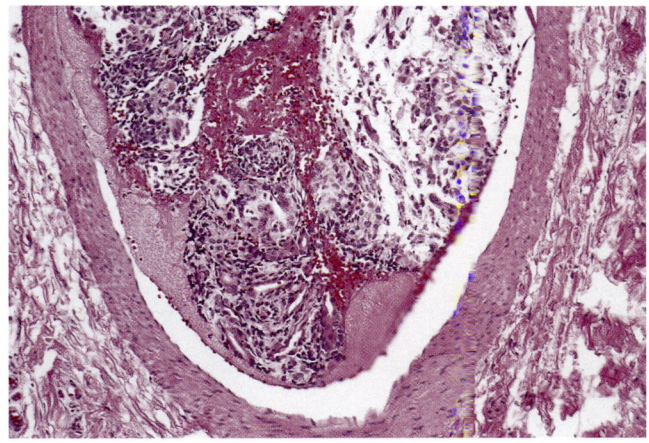

FIG. 1-53. Intravenous extension by carcinoma ex pleomorphic adenoma of parotid gland.

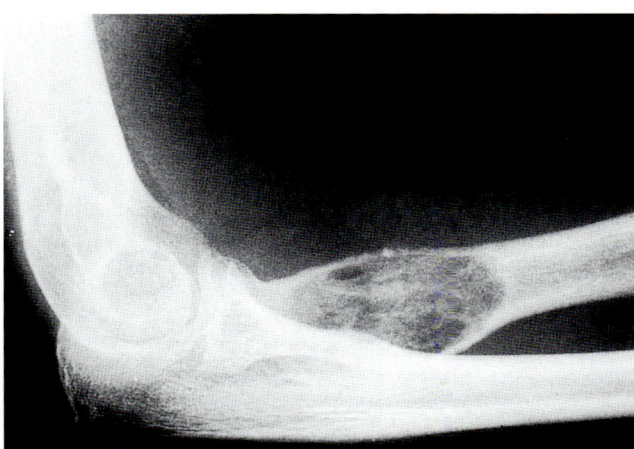

FIG. 1-54. Metastatic carcinoma ex pleomorphic adenoma in ulnar bone.

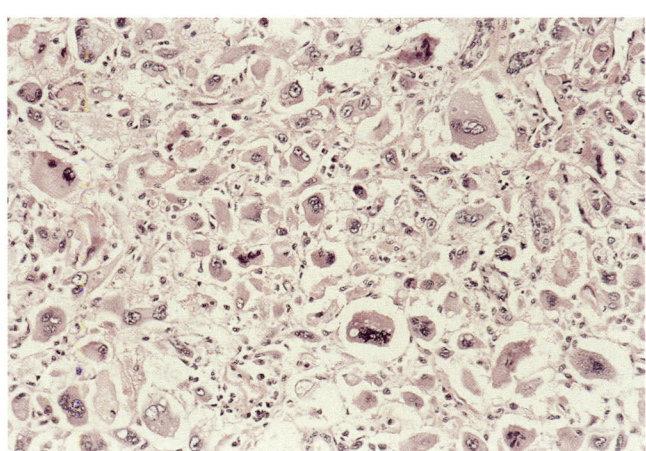

FIG. 1-55. High-grade carcinoma ex pleomorphic adenoma.

True Malignant Mixed Tumor (Carcinosarcoma, Sarcomatoid Carcinoma)

These tumors are characterized by the presence of both malignant epithelial and stromal components. They tend to be diffusely infiltrative and are refractory to treatment other than complete extirpation. The epithelial component may demonstrate a variety of characteristics, including both squamous carcinoma and adenocarcinoma. The stromal malignant component most frequently shows chondrosarcoma, but osteosarcoma and other spindle cell sarcomas may occur.

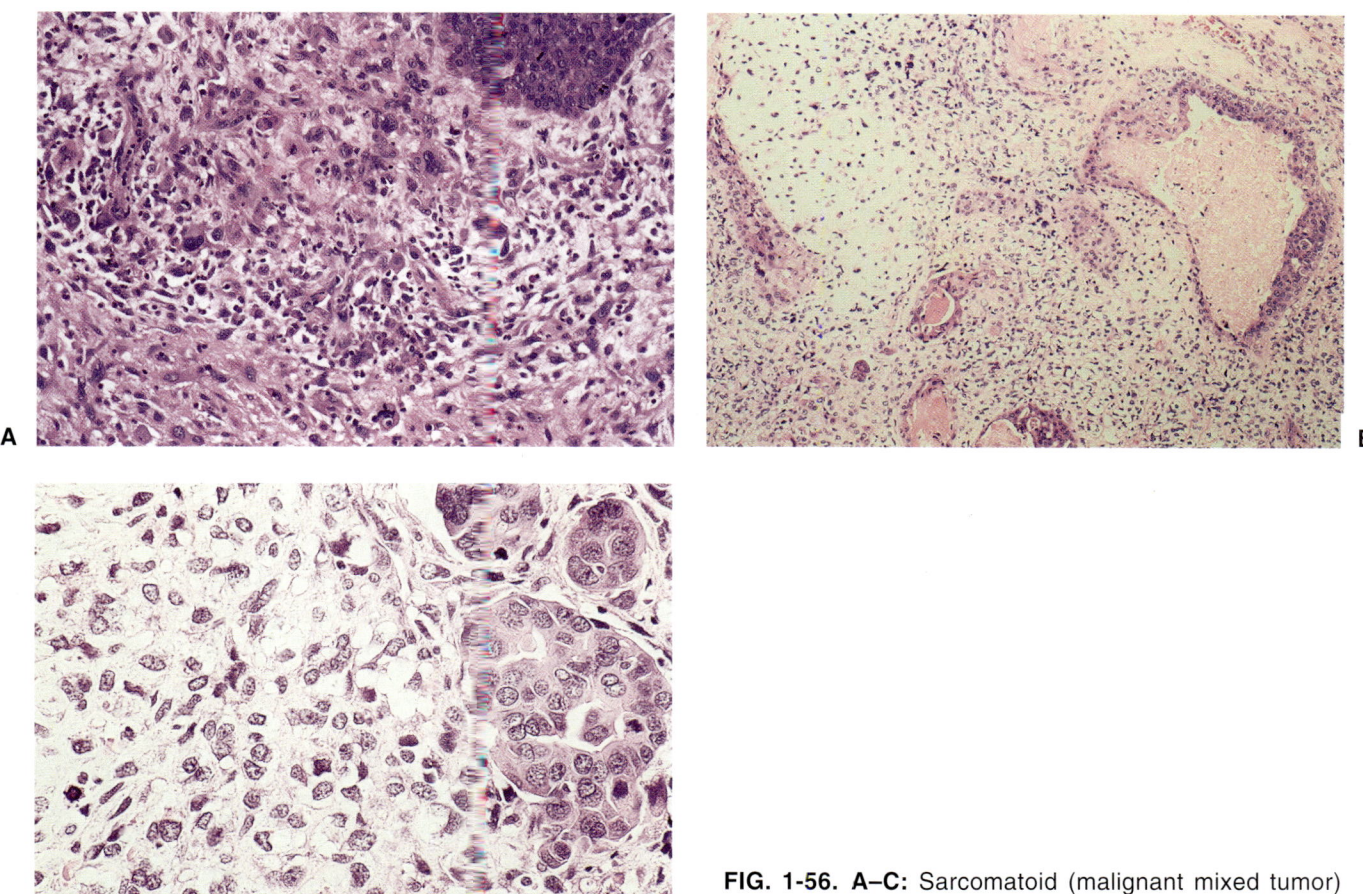

FIG. 1-56. A–C: Sarcomatoid (malignant mixed tumor) carcinoma of parotid gland.

Adenoid Cystic Carcinoma

Adenoid cystic carcinoma is the second most common malignant salivary gland tumor. Its clinical course is frequently marked by multiple local recurrences and, not infrequently, distant metastases. Its propensity for perineural invasion contributes greatly to the difficulty of achieving an adequate initial resection. The propensity for perineural invasion leads also to the not infrequent problem of intracranial extension of tumor along the course of cranial nerves.

The malignant cell in adenoid cystic carcinoma is a small (7 to 10 μm), hyperchromatic, "basaloid" cell with scanty, pale-staining cytoplasm. These cells demonstrate a variety of growth patterns, including cribriform, tubular, and solid. The histologic grade of the tumor can be low (tubuloductal architecture), intermediate (classic cribriform or "cylindromatous" appearance), or high (solid growth pattern). Mixtures of these patterns are common. The cribriform pattern is the most frequent and easily recognized. The malignant cells are arranged around small microcystic spaces filled with pale blue mucinous material, which represents reduplicated basal lamina. Mitoses vary in number and may be difficult to find at times.

The solid type demonstrates clustered cords of atypical cells forming syncytia, or islands, without microcystic spaces. The presence of reduplicated basal lamina can be demonstrated in the intercellular spaces with special stains and is a constant characteristic of the tubular and cribriform-cylindromatous types. The myoepithelial component is scant to absent in the solid adenoid cystic carcinoma, and the basement membrane is difficult to define.

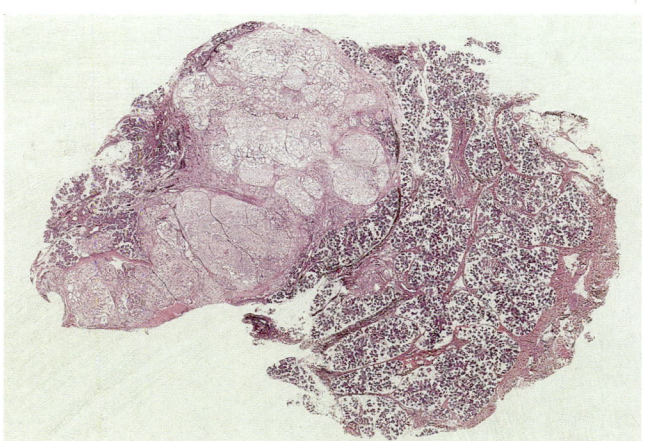

FIG. 1-57. Adenoid cystic carcinoma of parotid gland.

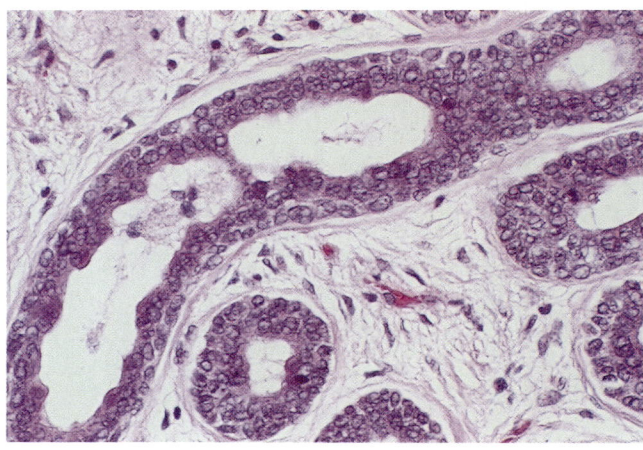

FIG. 1-58. Tubular adenoid cystic carcinoma (grade 1).

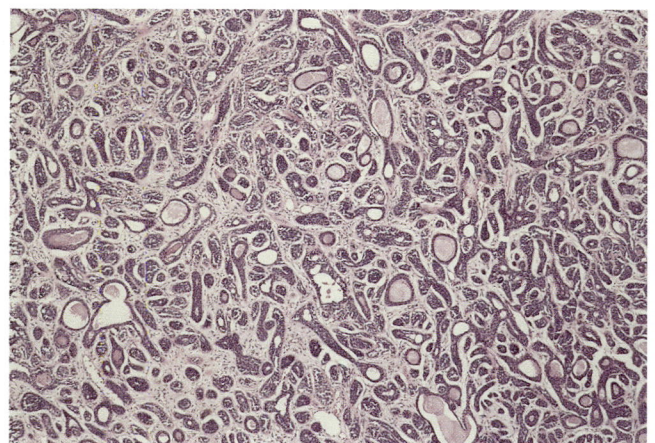

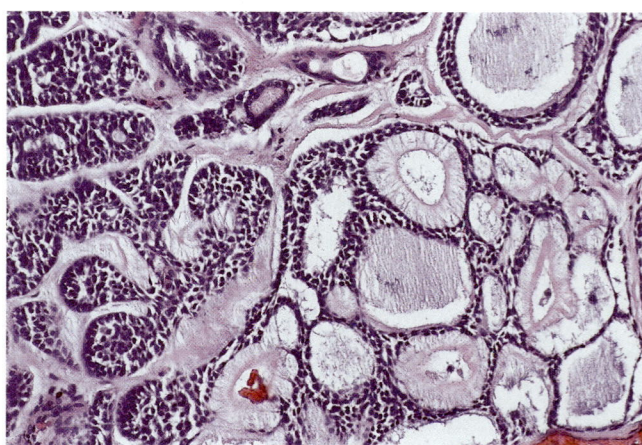

FIG. 1-59. A,B: Cribriform and cylindromatous adenoid cystic carcinoma.

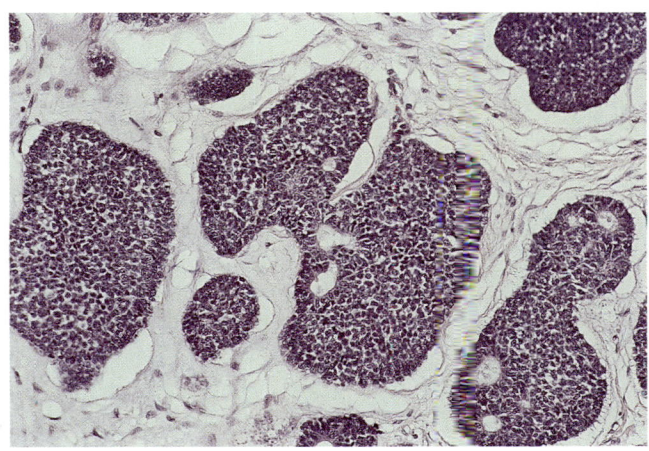 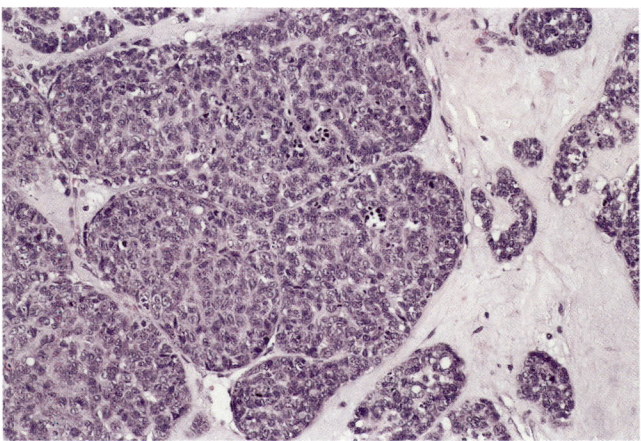

FIG. 1-60. A,B High-grade (grade 3; solid) adenoid cystic carcinoma.

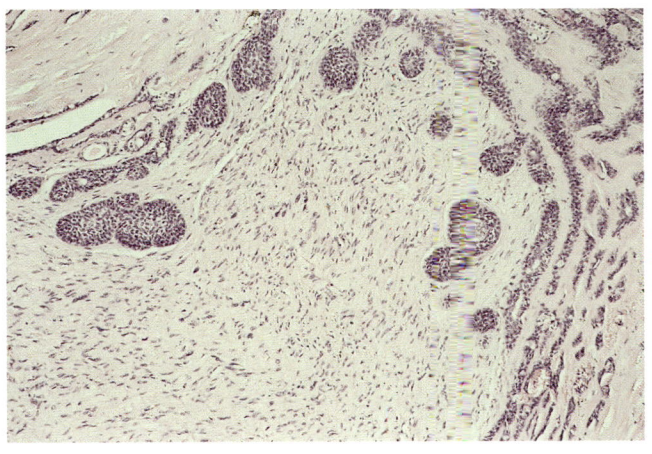

FIG. 1-61. Perineural and intraneural invasion by an adenoid cystic carcinoma.

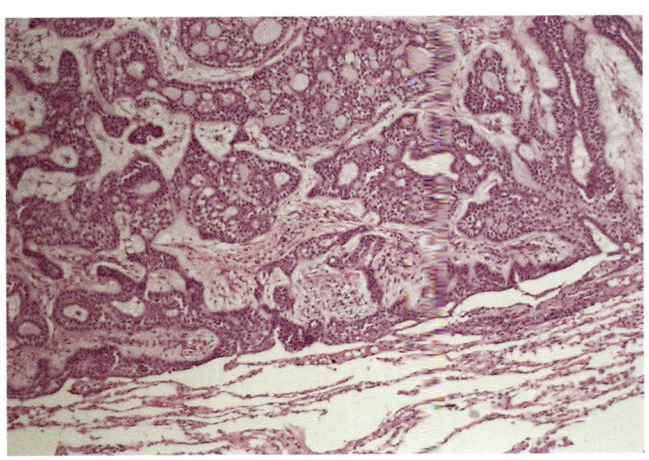 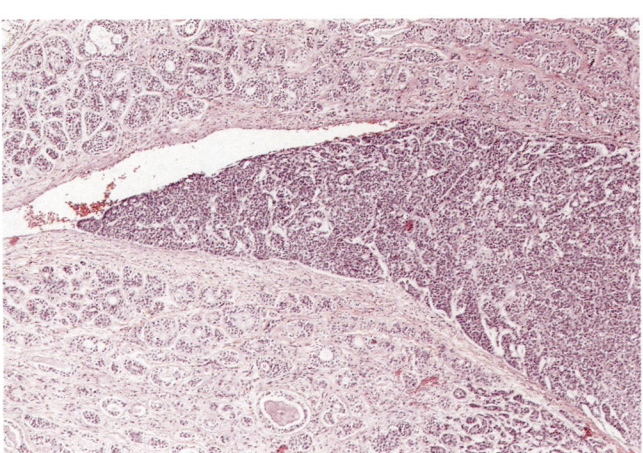

FIG. 1-62. A: Metastatic adenoid cystic carcinoma in lung. **B:** Adenoid cystic carcinoma invading large vein.

Polymorphous Low-grade Adenocarcinoma (Terminal Duct Adenocarcinoma)

This lesion involves the minor salivary glands almost exclusively, especially those of the oral cavity, with a predilection for the palate. Perineural invasion is a prominent feature, as is an "Indian filing" pattern of growth, but appear to have no prognostic significance. The malignant cells are typically arranged in a variety of growth patterns, including tubular, cystic, trabecular, and occasionally papillary. The tumors are biologically low-grade, although those with a papillary component possess a modest metastatic capability.

Mitoses are uncommon. Associated with the epithelial cells is an exuberant production of extracellular mucinous material, resembling pleomorphic adenoma. Unlike pleomorphic adenomas, these tumors do not demonstrate fibrous pseudoencapsulation, and infiltration around vascular and neural structures will be present. It is important not to confuse this tumor with adenoid cystic carcinoma or carcinoma ex pleomorphic adenoma, as these belong to significantly worse prognostic groups.

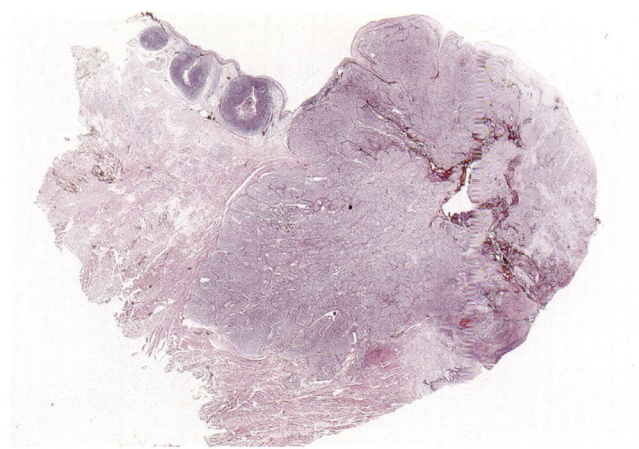

FIG. 1-63. Terminal duct adenocarcinoma of base of tongue.

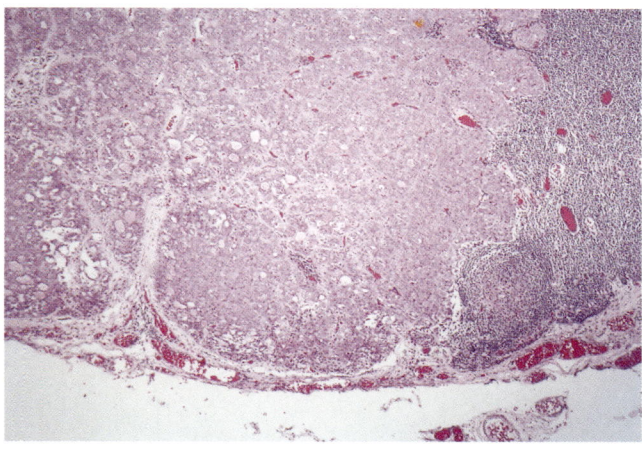

FIG. 1-65. Rare metastasis of terminal duct adenocarcinoma in a cervical lymph node. This usually occurs when the carcinoma shows a preponderance of papillary architecture.

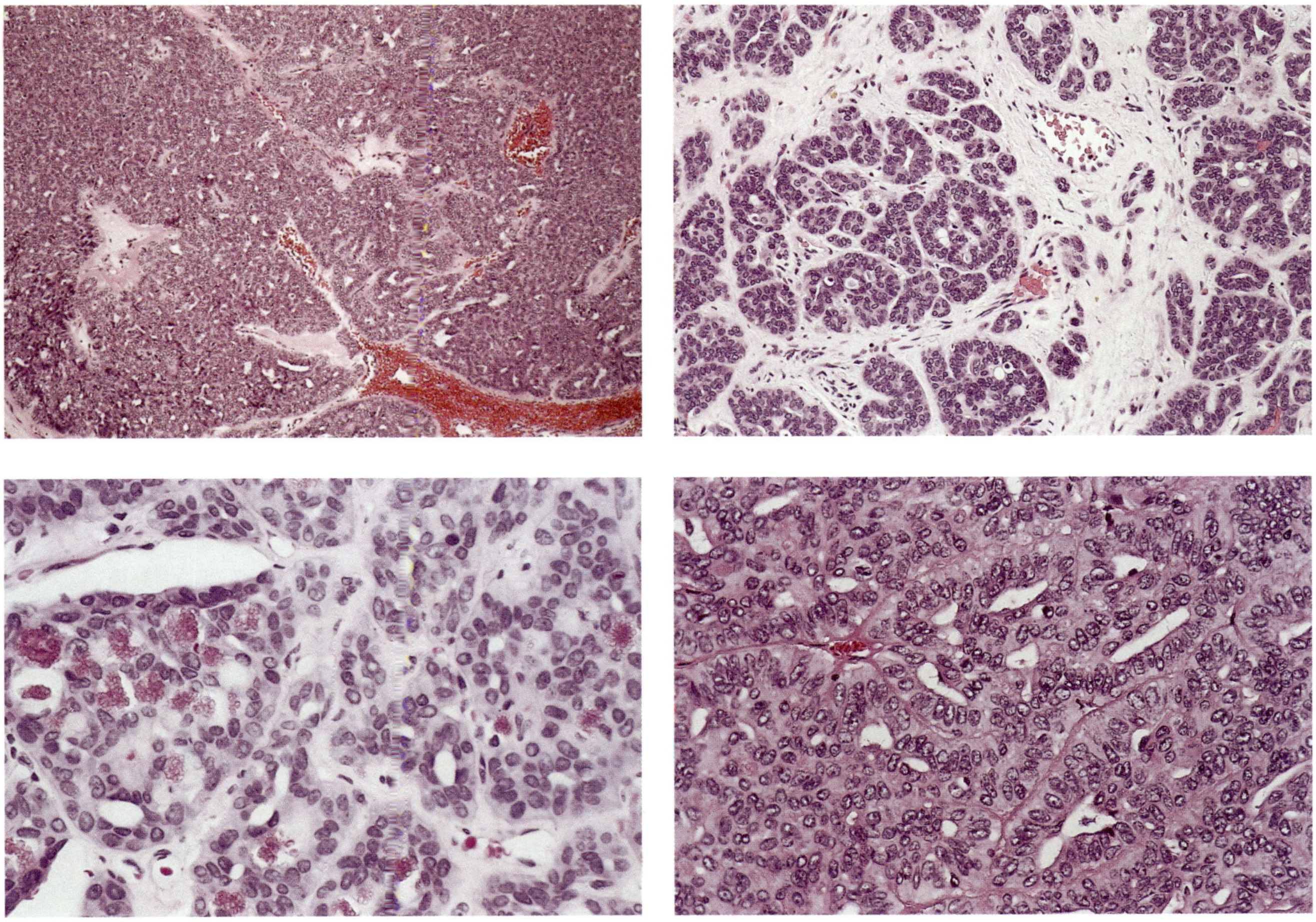

FIG. 1-64. A–D: Terminal duct adenocarcinoma of palate with its characteristic small ducts, some with luminal crystals (C).

Epimyoepithelial Carcinoma

The epimyoepithelial carcinoma is predominately a parotid malignancy and is biologically intermediate-grade. Its classic histologic appearance is that of a biphasic neoplasm with optically clear cells or spindle forms of the myoepithelial elements.

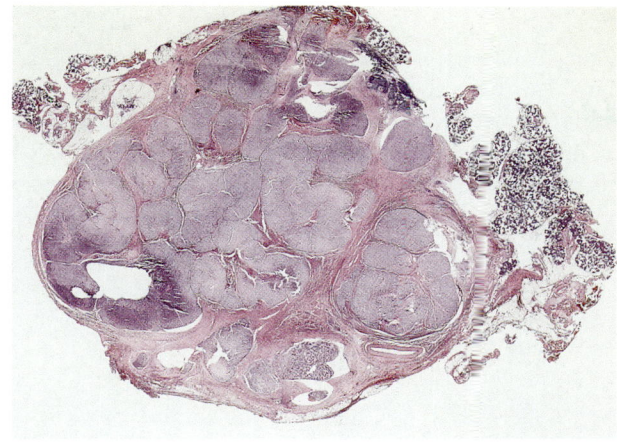

FIG. 1-66. Epimyoepithelial cell carcinoma of parotid gland. Note the typical lobular growth pattern.

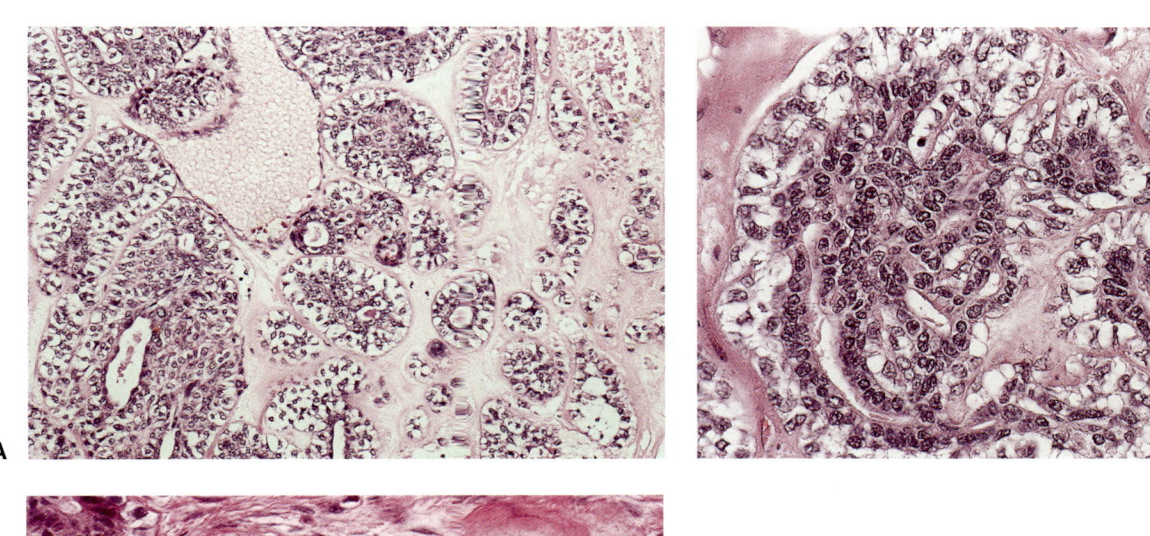

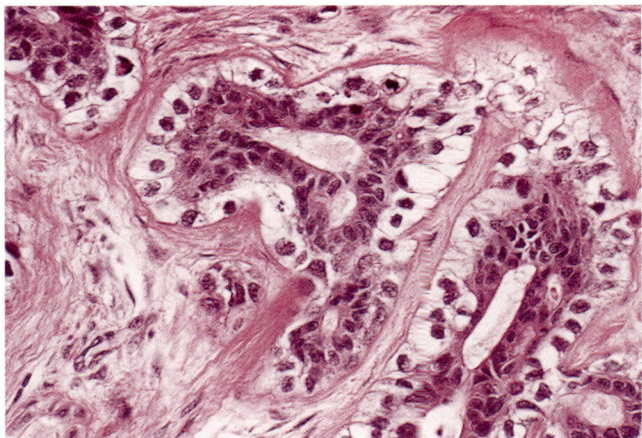

FIG. 1-67. A–C: Epimyoepithelial cell carcinoma in its classic biphasic (epithelial ductal and myoepithelial clear cell) appearance.

Salivary Duct Carcinoma

Even though the term adenocarcinoma can be applied to essentially all salivary malignancies, adenocarcinomas that can be recognized as such but not be subclassified in any glandular organ are uncommon. They arise from excretory ducts or major ducts and are devoid of myoepithelial cells. The salivary duct carcinoma is a prime example. Many salivary duct carcinomas look much like ductal carcinomas of the breast. They are always high-grade and are the most common type of carcinoma arising in a pleomorphic adenoma when not arising *de novo*.

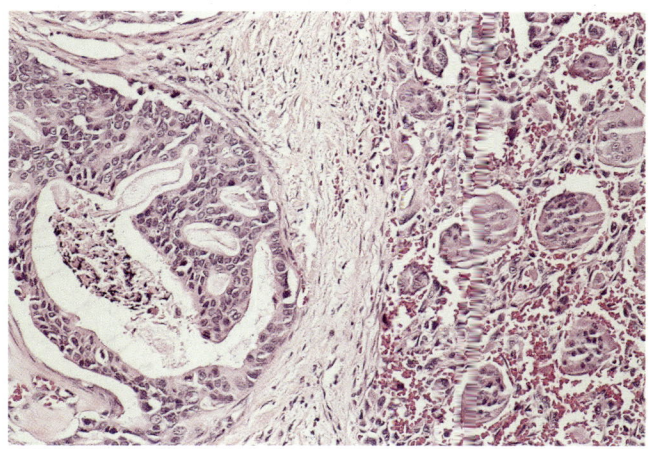

FIG. 1-68. Salivary duct (high-grade) carcinoma of the parotid gland. This example also shows an associated proliferation of osteoclast-like cells.

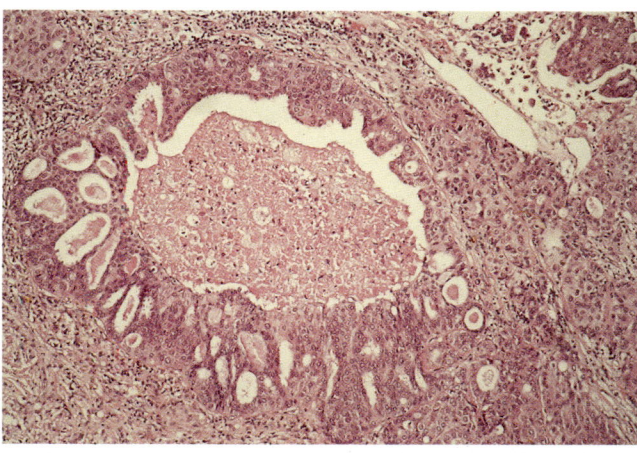

FIG. 1-69. Salivary duct carcinoma manifesting a close resemblance to mammary duct carcinoma, including comedonecrosis.

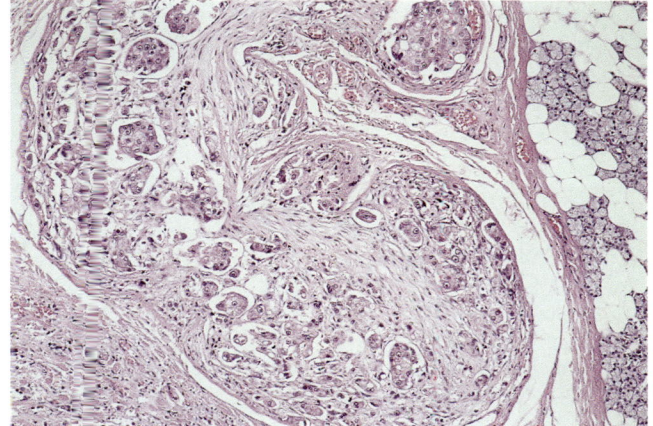

FIG. 1-70. Facial nerve branch extensively invaded by salivary duct carcinoma.

HISTOLOGY OF NONNEOPLASTIC LESIONS

Lymphoepithelial Lesion, Sialosis

Enlargement of the salivary glands, particularly the parotid glands, can reflect systemic and metabolic disorders. Prominent among these are Sjögren's syndrome and sialadenosis (sialosis).

The salivary gland manifestation of the immunologic exocrinopathy known as Sjögren's syndrome is the lymphoepithelial lesion. A diagnosis of Sjögren's syndrome cannot be made on histologic grounds alone, as the syndrome is a clinical-immunologic disorder. The lymphoepithelial lesion, although characteristic, is not pathognomonic of Sjögren's syndrome. With progressive lymphoid cell infiltration, the affected salivary gland is converted to a parenchyma-poor lymphoid lesion in which metaplastic epimyoepithelial islands are seen. Labial biopsy specimens may reflect the disease and how severe it is. Sites in the oral cavity can also be affected.

Sustained antigenic stimulation and salivary duct-acinar destruction with lymphoid cell proliferation can eventually develop into either low-grade B-cell lymphoma (mucosa-associated lymphoid tissue, or MALT) or higher-grade lymphoma in the salivary glands and/or lymph nodes.

Sialadenosis is most often a bilateral parotid enlargement and is the consequence of parasympathetic nerve imbalance, malnutrition, alcoholism, bulimia, diabetes mellitus, and other systemic disorders. Secretory granule-loaded acinar cells are typical of sialadenosis. In end-stage disease, only an acinar cell-depleted and fibrotic salivary gland may be seen.

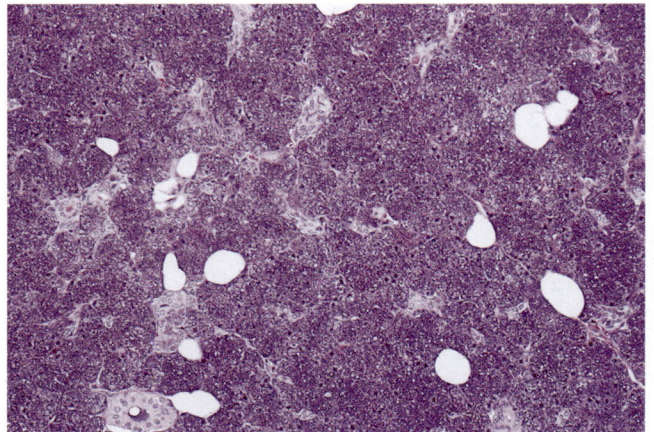 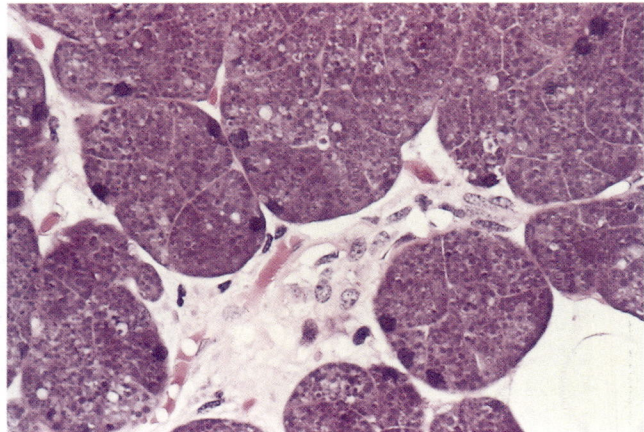

FIG. 1-71. A,B: Sialosis of parotid gland. Swollen acinar cells are filled with secretory product.

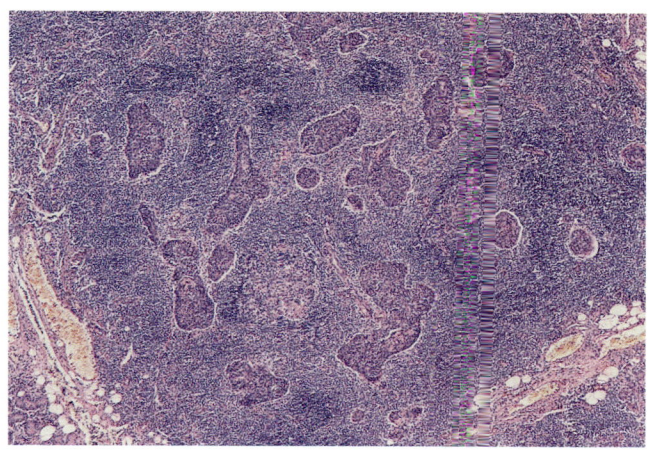

FIG. 1-72. Lymphoepithelial lesion of parotid gland. Epimyoepithelial islands in lymphoid cell-replaced parenchyma.

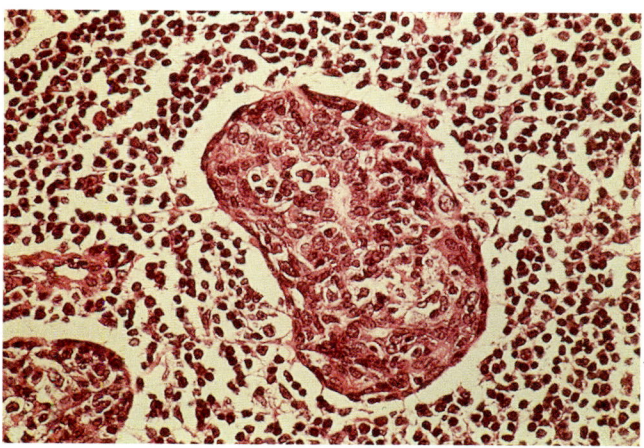

FIG. 1-73. Epimyoepithelial island in lymphoepithelial lesion.

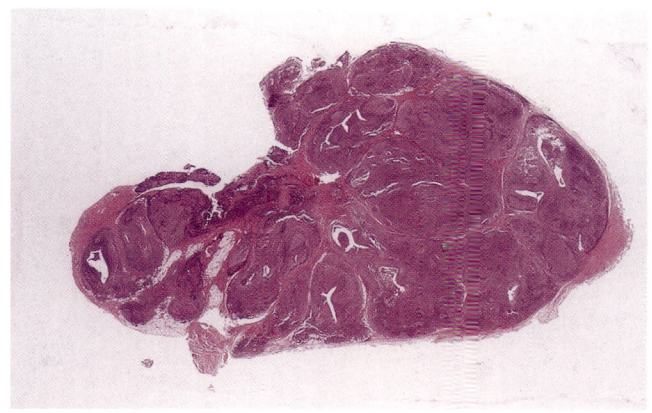

FIG. 1-74. Nearly end-stage lymphoepithelial lesion with almost complete replacement of parotid parenchyma by lymphoid tissue.

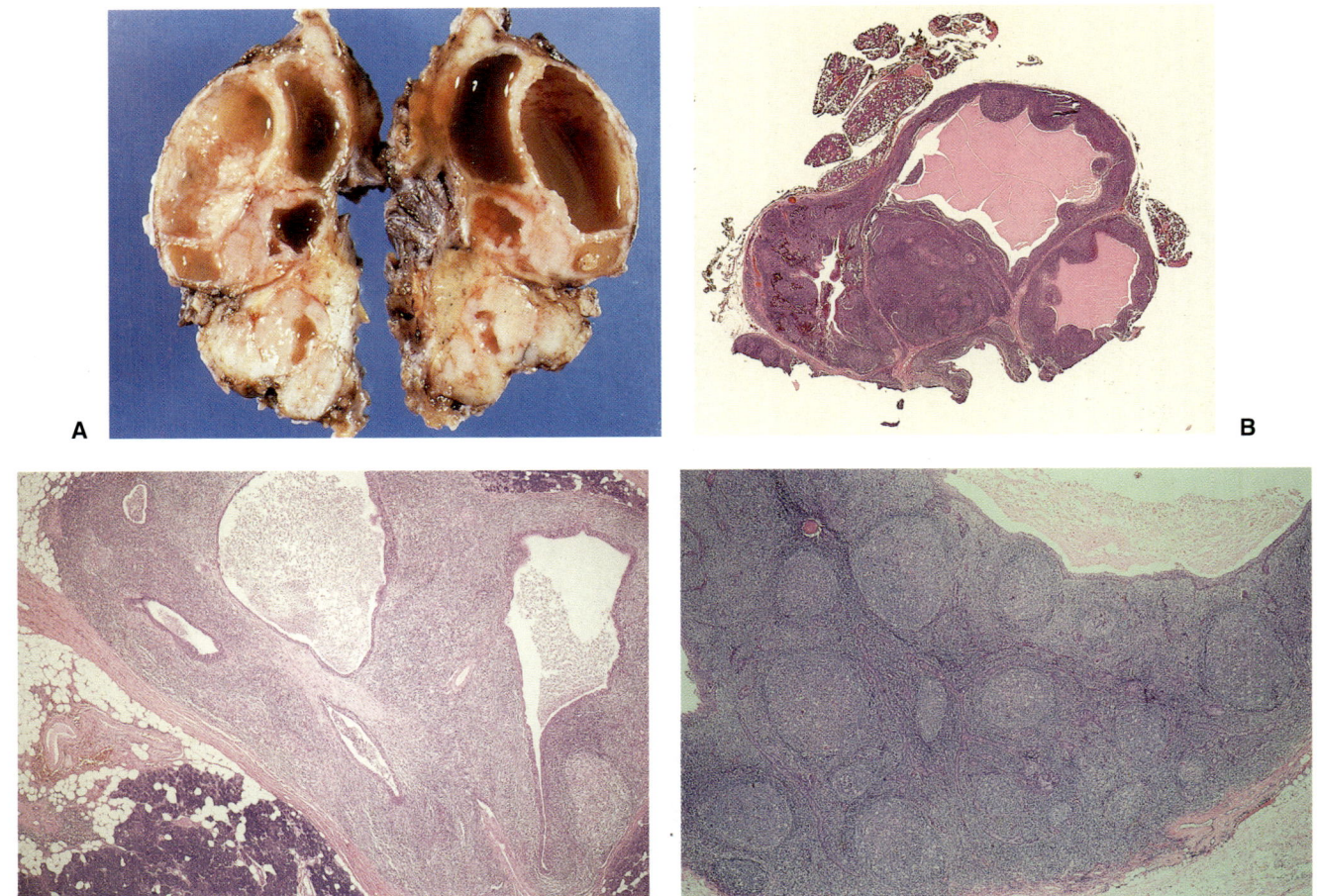

FIG. 1-75. A–D: Lymphoepithelial cysts from HIV-positive patients. Note the associated follicular lymphoid hyperplasia in D.

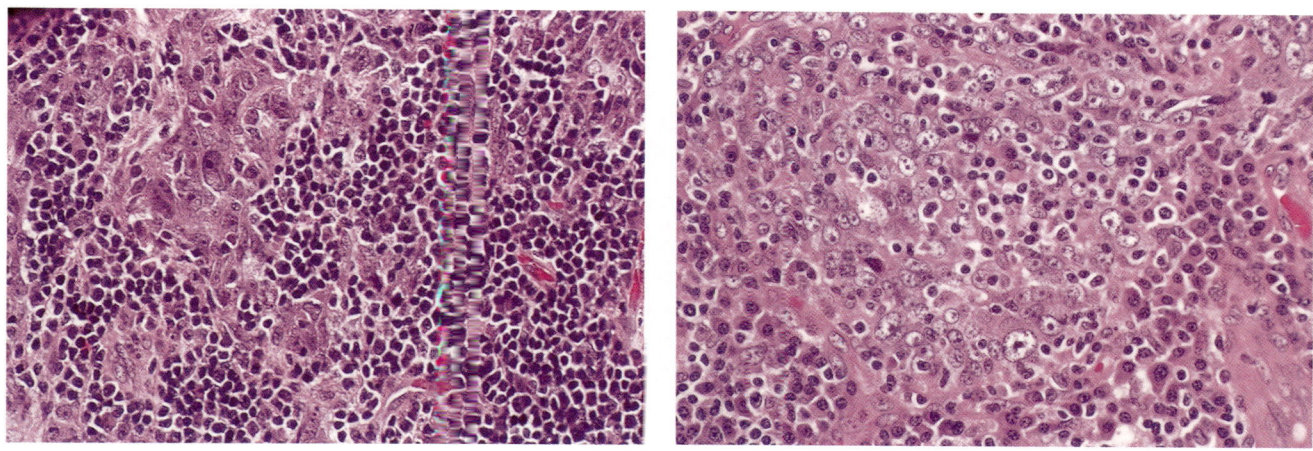

FIG. 1-76. A,B: Lymphoepithelial carcinoma of the parotid gland, also known as undifferentiated carcinoma with lymphoid stroma.

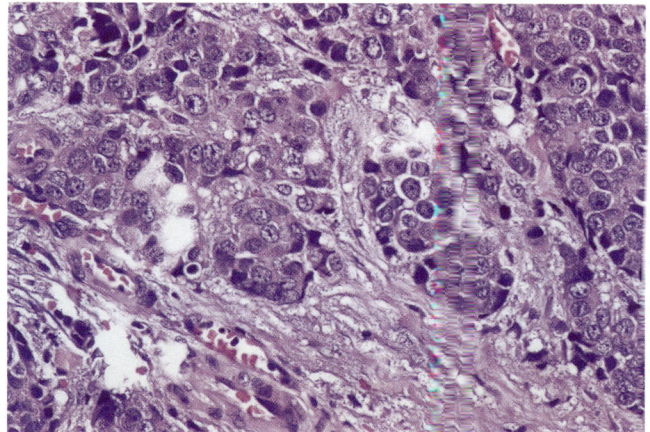

FIG. 1-77. Undifferentiated carcinoma, no neuroendocrine, of the parotid gland.

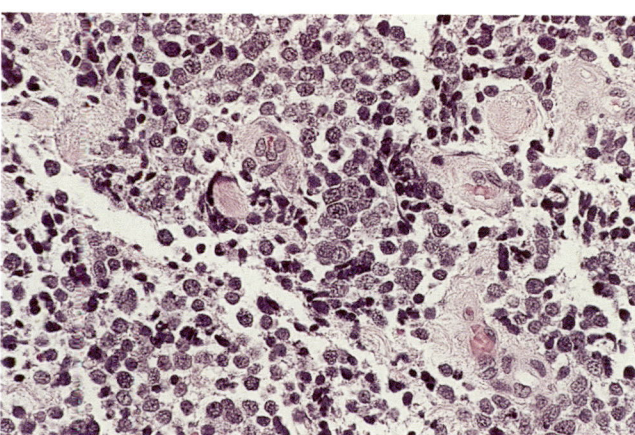

FIG. 1-78. Neuroendocrine carcinoma of the parotid gland.

Sjögren's Syndrome

Presentation

Sjögren's syndrome is an autoimmune disease characterized by lymphocyte-mediated destruction of the exocrine glands, which leads to xerostomia and keratoconjunctivitis sicca.

Histology

The histologic equivalent of Sjögren's syndrome is lymphoepithelial sialadenopathy; without clinical reference, it is nonspecific. The parotid gland in Sjögren's syndrome is at risk for the development of lymphoma. The epimyoepithelial islands can rarely be the origin of a carcinoma.

Mucocele/Ranula

Mucocele and ranula are related lesions, differing only in location and potential size. Each is a mucous extravasation phenomenon and therefore a pseudocystic lesion. Mucoceles have a predilection for the lips, and ranulae for the floor of mouth and soft tissue of the neck (plunging ranula). The plunging or cervical ranula originates in the sublingual glands; mucoceles originate in minor salivary glands.

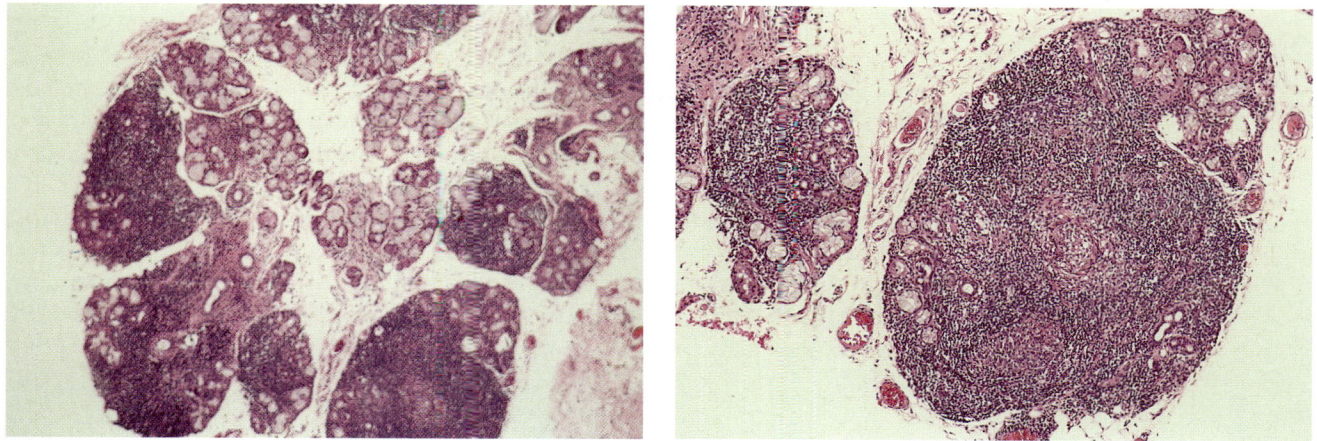

FIG. 1-79. A,B: Labial (lip) biopsy specimen from a patient with Sjögren's syndrome.

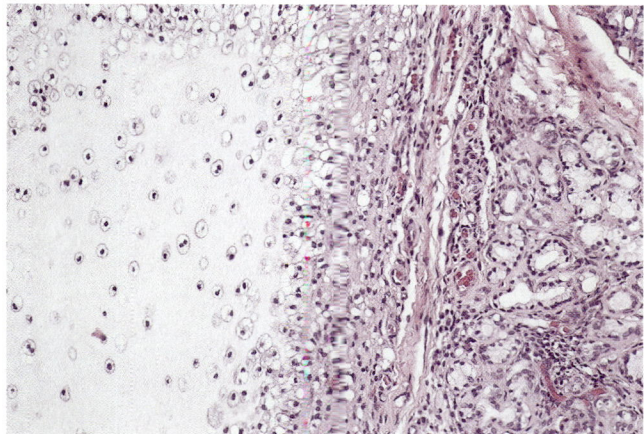

FIG. 1-80. Mucocele of the lip.

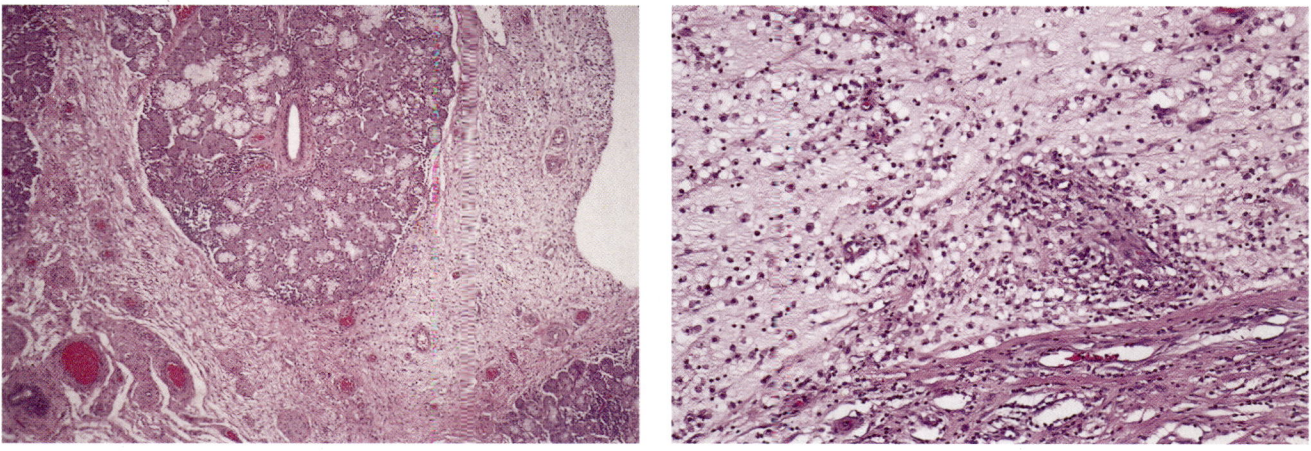

FIG. 1-81. A,B: Cervical (plunging) ranula. The ranula may be exterior to the submandibular gland and does not arise from the gland.

Necrotizing Sialometaplasia; Sialolithiasis

Two nonneoplastic oral lesions that simulate malignancies can be likened to "a sheep in wolf's clothing." One is a glandular hyperplasia, usually of the palate or buccal mucosa, called adenomatous hyperplasia. The other, which is far more troublesome in regard to differential diagnosis, is necrotizing sialometaplasia. Necrotizing sialometaplasia, although most noteworthy in the oral cavity and palate, can occur in any salivary gland tissue. In extraoral sites, the lesion nearly always follows tissue injury, usually an iatrogenic infarct. In the oral cavity, the cause is more nebulous but still has a vascular basis. Squamous metaplasia of ducts and acini in various stages of development is the prominent and most histologically disconcerting feature. Preservation of the minor salivary gland lobular architecture is very important in the differential diagnosis.

A B C D

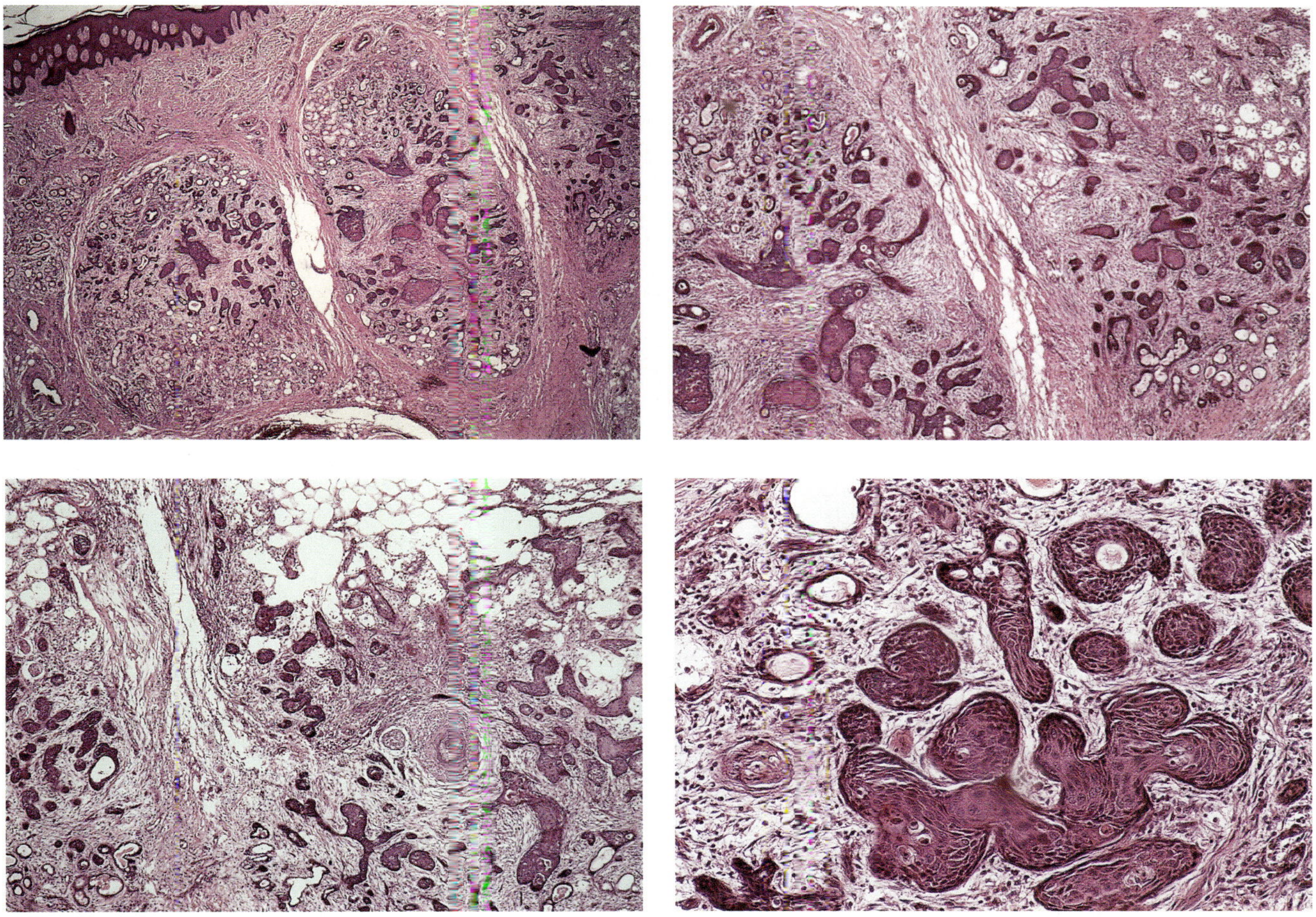

FIG. 1-82. A–D: Necrotizing sialometaplasia of palate. Note preserved lobular architecture and also the occluded artery in C.

A B

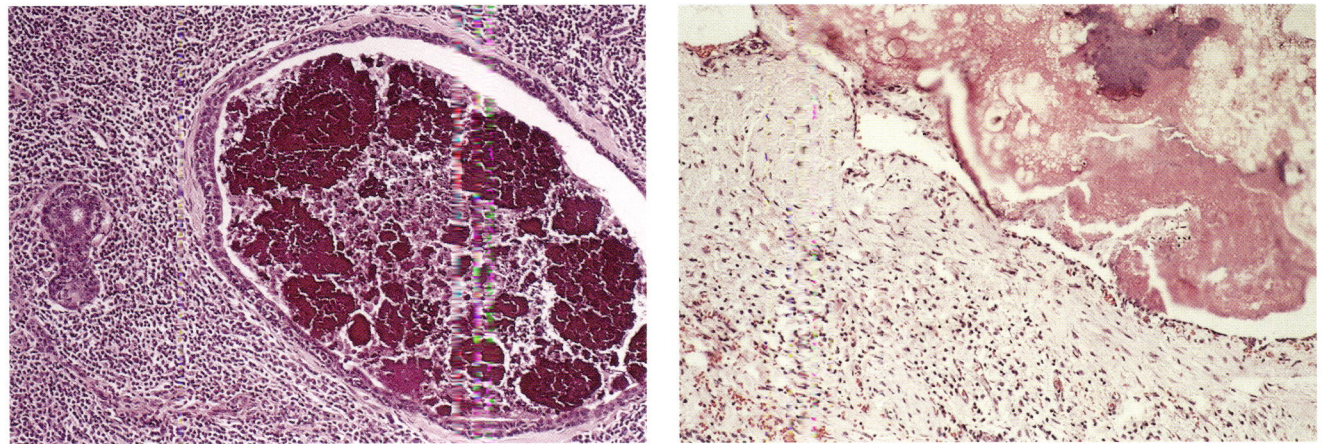

FIG. 1-83. A,B: Sialoliths in submandibular gland ducts.

Sialadenitis

Inflammatory disease (exclusive of ganulomatous disease) of the major salivary glands is nearly always duct-based, with a varying degree of immunologic modulation. The submandibular gland is considered to be more predisposed to inflammatory disorders, with or without sialolithiasis. Chronic, recurrent sialadenitis may be associated with considerable morbidity and replacement of the acinar parenchyma by fibrosis. The so-called "Küttner tumor" of the submandibular gland is a pronounced example of "tumorlike fibrosis."

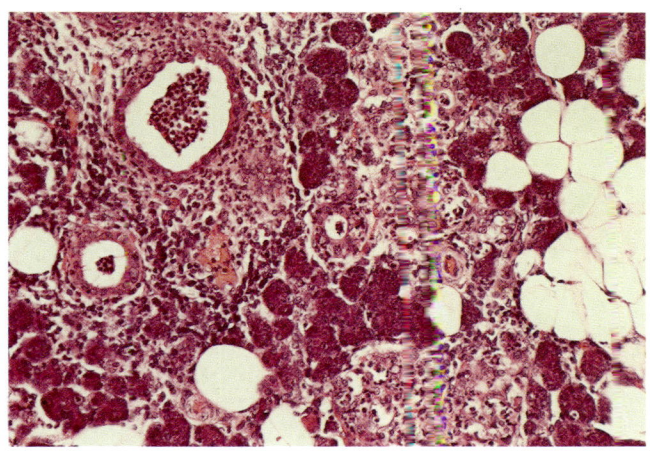

FIG. 1-84. Acute sialadenitis of parotid gland. Acute inflammatory exudate appears within ducts and parenchyma.

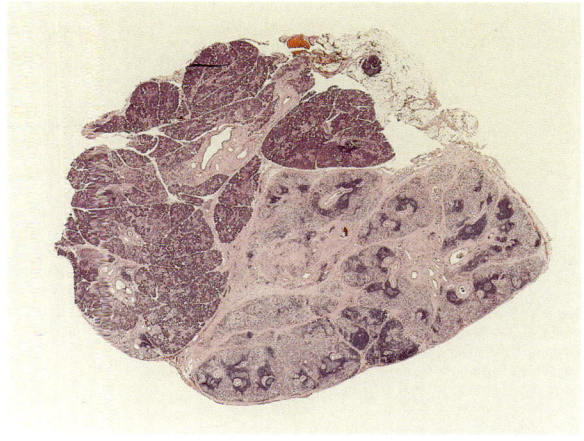

FIG. 1-85. Chronic sialadenitis of the submandibular gland.

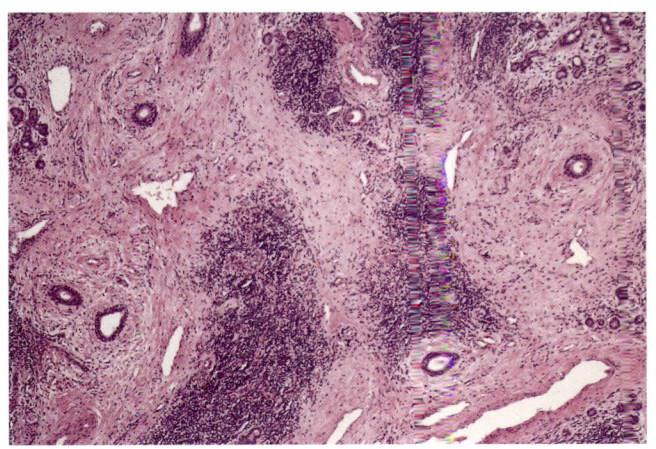
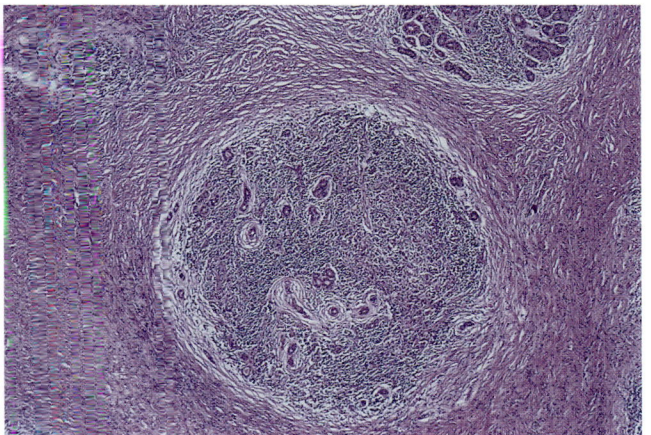

FIG. 1-86. A,B: Chronic sclerosing sialadenitis (Küttner tumor) of submandibular gland.

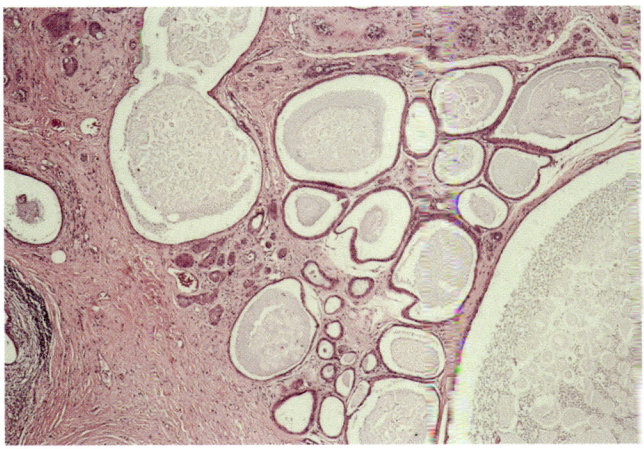
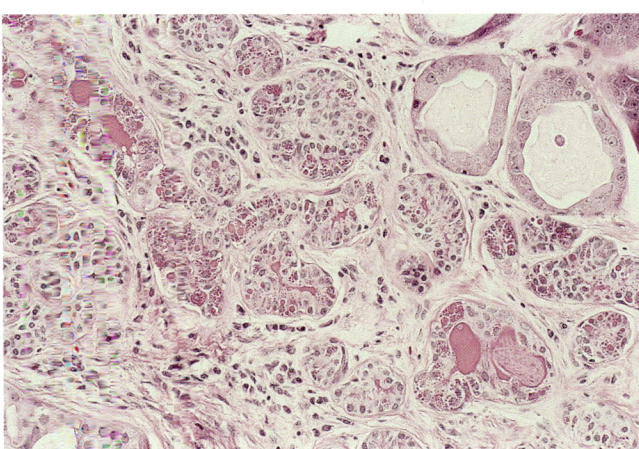

FIG. 1-87. A,B: Chronic recurrent sialadenitis of parotid gland.

2

Thyroid Gland

THYROGLOSSAL DUCT CYST

Presentation

This lesion presents as a midline neck mass that is frequently cystic on examination and occasionally secondarily infected.

Pathophysiology

Failure of complete descent of the thyroid anlage can result in deposition of thyroid tissue anywhere from the base of the tongue to the thyroid bed itself. Lingual thyroid is the presence of thyroid at the base of the tongue, but the most common defect in migration is the thyroglossal duct cyst. The lesion is intimately associated with the hyoid bone.

Histology

The lining varies from simple to stratified squamous and respiratory epithelium but may also demonstrate other types. The cyst usually contains keratin debris and may be complex in its structure. Within the wall of the cyst, one should find residual elements of thyroid tissue. These thyroid remnants can give rise to carcinoma, usually papillary.

HASHIMOTO'S THYROIDITIS

Presentation

Hashimoto's thyroiditis may present as a unilateral or bilateral thyroid mass in the lower neck.

Pathophysiology

This is an autoimmune disease of cryptogenic etiology.

Histology

There is a lymphocytic infiltration and oncocytic cellular change with progressive destruction of the gland over time.

GRAVES' DISEASE

Presentation

Graves' disease may present with enlargement of the thyroid gland or with secondary signs, such as exophthalmos.

Pathophysiology

This also is an autoimmune disease, but it leads to glandular hyperfunction.

Histology

The lobular architecture is retained, but with a prominent vascular congestion and follicular hyperplasia. The follicular cells are columnar. Colloid is scant, with scalloping at the periphery.

MULTINODULAR GOITER

Presentation

Multinodular goiter may present as a unilateral or bilateral mass in the lower neck.

Pathophysiology

This benign enlargement of the thyroid is felt to result from iodine deficiency or impairment of uptake. Multiple nodules are usually present within the gland, but there may be only one, or one nodule may predominate.

Histology

Histologically, there are benign colloid nodules of widely varying size.

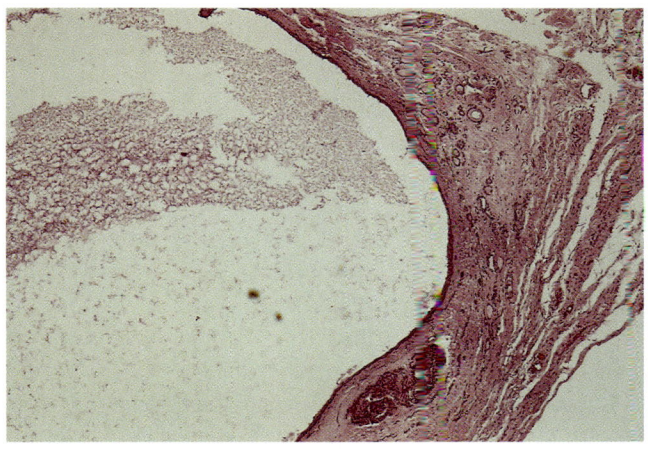

FIG. 2-1. Thyroglossal duct cyst. Nodules of ectopic thyroid tissue may be seen in the wall of the cyst.

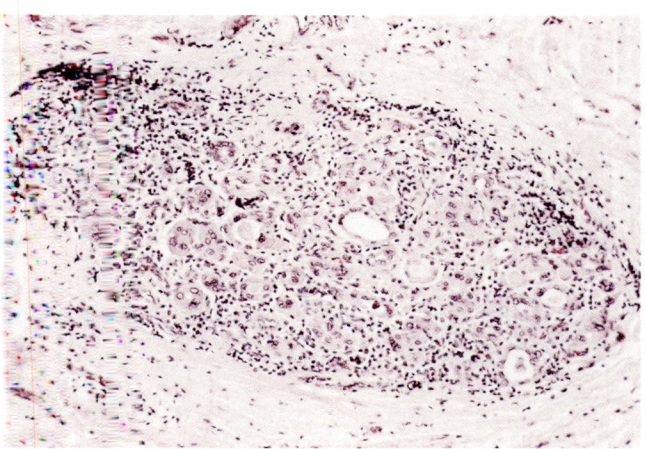

FIG. 2-2. Chronic Hashimoto's thyroiditis.

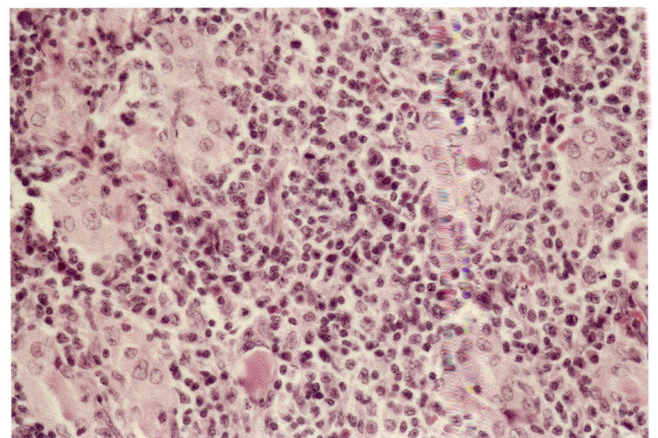

FIG. 2-3. Hashimoto's thyroiditis.

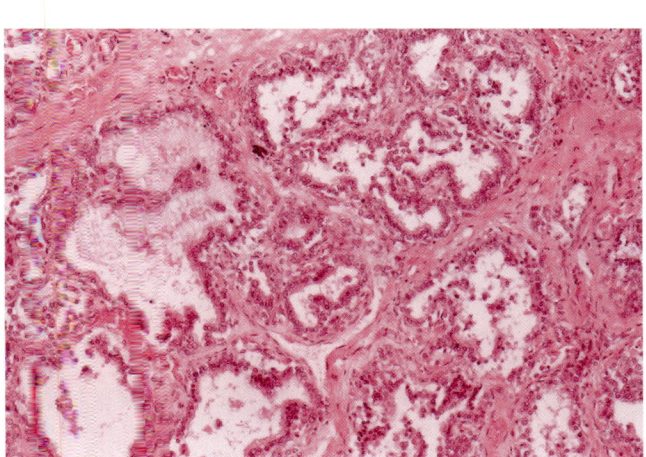

FIG. 2-4. Graves' disease.

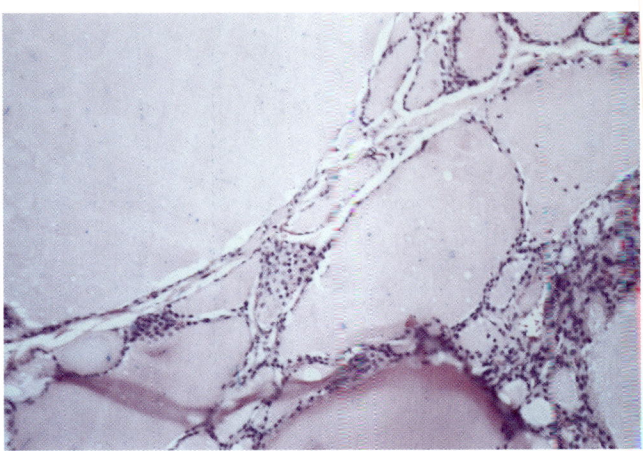

FIG. 2-5. Benign adenomatous goiter.

PAPILLARY THYROID CARCINOMA

Presentation

Most papillary carcinomas present as a thyroid mass, but some cases present with cervical adenopathy (metastasis).

Pathophysiology

Papillary carcinoma is the most common neoplasm of the thyroid, accounting for 75% of all thyroid malignancies and 80% to 90% of radiation-induced neoplasms. The tumor is classified as occult (<1.5 cm), intrathyroid, or extrathyroid. Occult neoplasms are found in 6% to 13% of autopsies in the United States. The peak incidence of this tumor is in the third to fourth decades; in contrast, the peak incidence of follicular carcinoma occurs later in adulthood. In 50% to 75% of cases, the tumor is multifocal. The incidence of regional metastases has been reported to be as high as 50%. The presence of regional metastasis increases the likelihood of local recurrence; however, it does not appear to affect survival. Although papillary carcinoma is four times more common in women, the prognosis is worse for men. In addition, extrathyroid spread and age above 40 years are associated with a worse prognosis. The most common site of distant metastasis is the lung. The relative frequency of papillary carcinoma is reported to be even higher in children than in adults. The mortality rate of this neoplasm is 1% to 10%. The tall cell variant has a worse prognosis.

Preoperative indicators of a poorer prognosis include age above 40 years, grade, extent, and size (AGES), as well as male sex. Some believe completeness of resection also affects prognosis, so that another prognostic scoring system is based on metastasis, age, completeness of resection, invasion, and sex (MACIS).

Histology

Histologically, there are papillary fronds of follicular cells with a fibrovascular core. Psammoma bodies may be present. The nuclei have been described as "Orphan Annie" because of their clear or nearly clear appearance; they are often grooved.

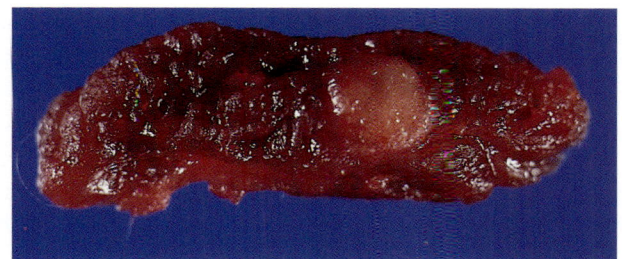

FIG. 2-6. Papillary carcinoma of the thyroid gland.

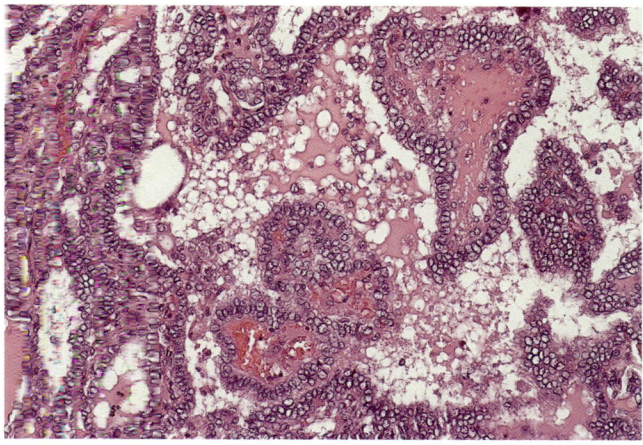

FIG. 2-7. Papillary carcinoma of the thyroid gland.

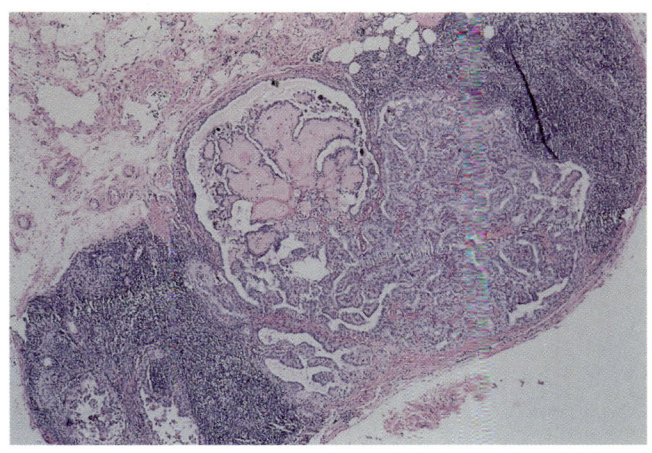

FIG. 2-8. Metastatic papillary carcinoma in cervical lymph node.

FOLLICULAR CARCINOMA

Presentation

Follicular carcinoma almost always presents as a thyroid mass.

Pathophysiology

Follicular carcinoma is the second most common thyroid neoplasm, accounting for 10% to 15% of all thyroid cancers. Peak incidence occurs in the fifth decade. Multiple foci are rarely seen in this disease. Malignancy is determined by vascular and capsular invasion. Like papillary carcinoma, this tumor occurs more commonly in women but has a poorer prognosis in men. Lymph node involvement is seen much less often in follicular than in papillary carcinoma, and its presence usually indicates a poor prognosis. Patients under 40 years of age are more frequently cured of their disease than are older patients.

Metastases occur via hematogenous spread, usually to lung, bone, and brain. Local recurrence of follicular carcinoma, unlike that of papillary cancer, is felt to be related directly to an increased mortality rate. The 10-year survival rate has been reported to be 43% to 70% by various authors.

Histology

Histologically, the tumor has a microfollicular or trabecular pattern with regular, small, round follicles. The criterion for malignancy is the demonstration of either capsular or vascular invasion. The latter carries a worse prognosis; most cases involve veins at or beyond the capsule.

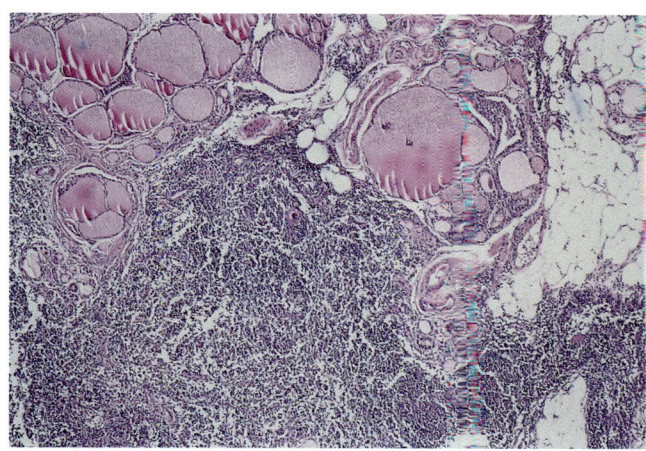

FIG. 2-9. Ectopic thyroid follicles in thymus gland.

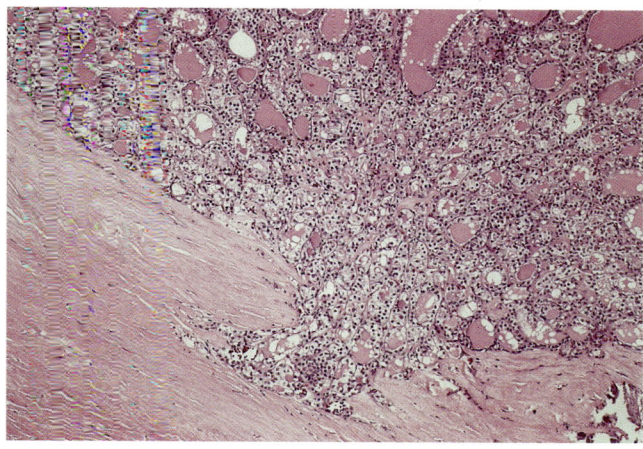

FIG. 2-10. Intracapsular extension by follicular thyroid carcinoma.

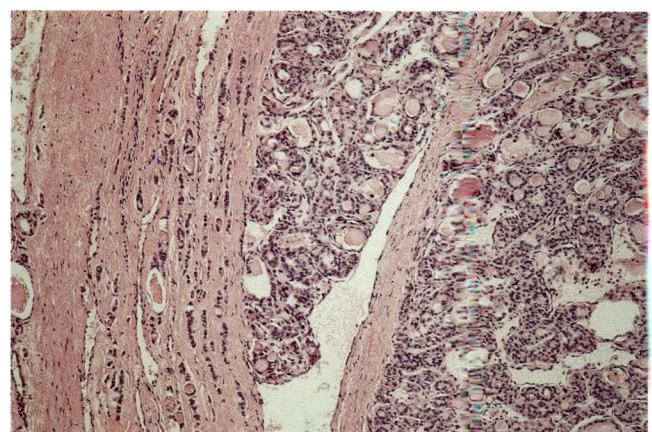
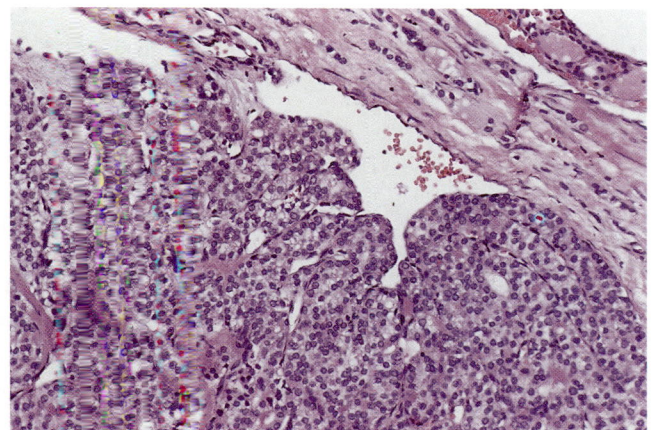

FIG. 2-11. A,B: Vascular invasion by follicular carcinoma.

FOLLICULAR VARIANT OF PAPILLARY CARCINOMA

Histologically, both follicles and papillae are present in most cases of papillary carcinoma. Some variants will have almost all follicles present in the primary tumor, with papillary features in the metastases. Most importantly, however, the ratio of follicles to papillae does not seem to have any effect on prognosis. These lesions behave clinically like pure papillary cancers. This is the so-called "Lindsay tumor." Clues that the tumor is truly a papillary variant include the presence of Orphan Annie nuclei and psammoma bodies.

HÜRTHLE CELL CARCINOMA

Pathophysiology

Hürthle cell (oxyphilic) tumors account for 5% to 6% of all thyroid neoplasms. They are considered to be a variant of follicular carcinoma but are thought to behave more aggressively. As with other follicular neoplasms, malignancy is determined by vascular and capsular invasion. Often, both lobes of the thyroid are involved. Because of the more invasive nature of this tumor, treatment should be aggressive.

Histology

Hürthle cell neoplasms are most often follicular in pattern, and the criteria for malignancy are the same as for follicular carcinoma or papillary carcinoma.

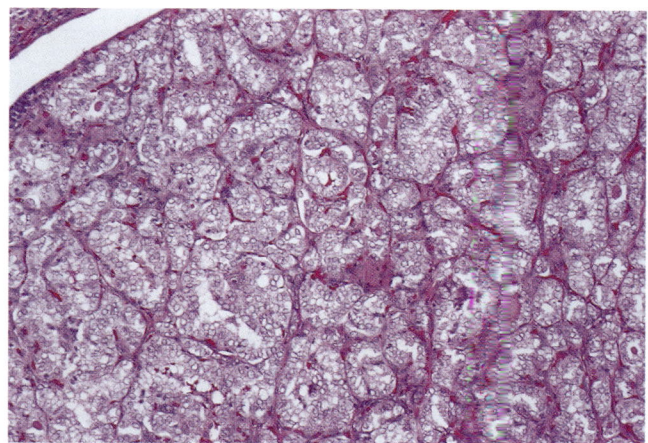

FIG. 2-12. Follicular variant of papillary carcinoma of the thyroid gland (Lindsay tumor).

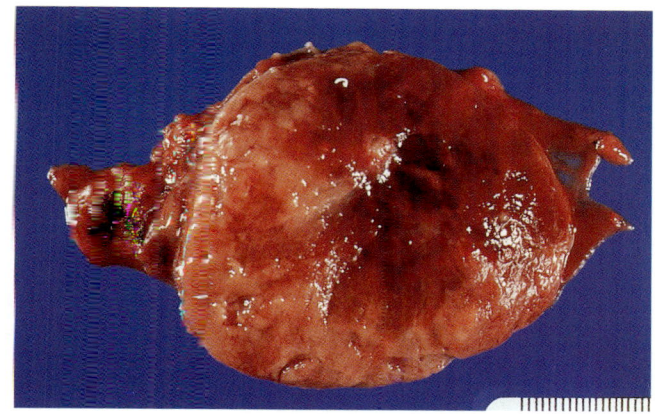

FIG. 2-13. Hürthle cell tumor of thyroid gland.

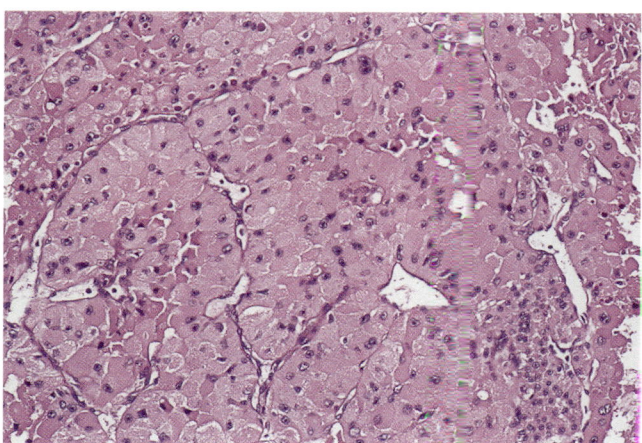

FIG. 2-14. A,B: Hürthle cell tumors of the thyroid gland.

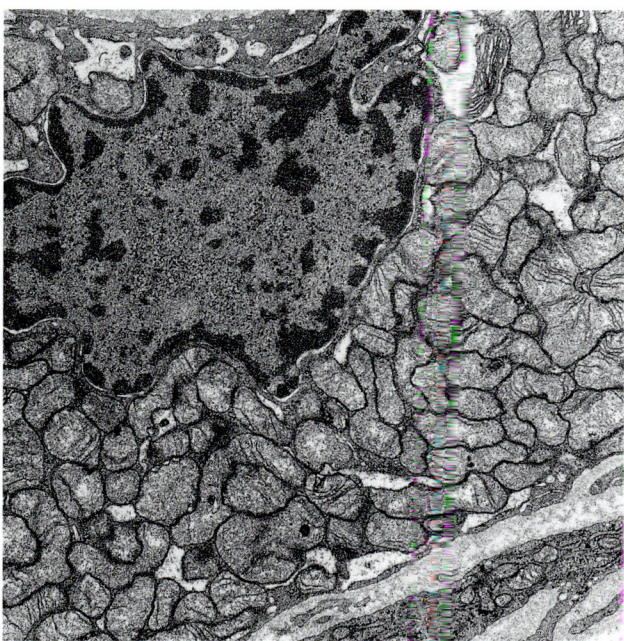

FIG. 2-15. Mitochondria-rich Hürthle cell as seen with the electron microscope.

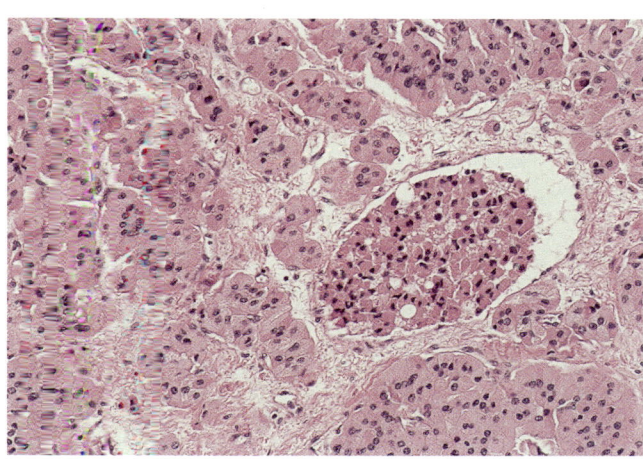

FIG. 2-16. Vascular invasion by a Hürthle cell carcinoma.

MEDULLARY CARCINOMA

Presentation

Most cases present as a thyroid mass.

Pathophysiology

Medullary carcinoma accounts for 5% to 10% of thyroid cancers. This tumor originates from nonepithelial C cells, derived from neuroectoderm. C cells secrete calcitonin, which can therefore be used as a tumor marker. Medullary carcinoma occurs in both sporadic and familial forms. The sporadic type comprises 70% to 90% of medullary cancers, and the familial type accounts for 10% to 30% of these tumors. The sporadic form, which is generally a unilateral nodule in an older patient (>50 years), has a poorer prognosis than its familial counterpart. The familial form is inherited as an autosomal dominant trait. This type can be part of a multiple endocrine adenomatosis syndrome. Multiple endocrine neoplasia (MEN) type IIA is characterized by medullary carcinoma, hyperparathyroidism, and pheochromocytoma. MEN type IIB includes medullary carcinoma, mucosal neuromas, pheochromocytoma, intestinal ganglioneuromas, and marfanoid habitus. The familial type is more likely to be multifocal, occurs in a younger population, and has a better prognosis. The familial type is also characterized by the presence of C-cell hyperplasia in other areas of the gland. More than 50% of patients have regional lymph node involvement, and in up to 50%, nodes are palpable on initial presentation. The presence of lymph node metastasis has an adverse effect on survival. Lymphatic spread is the major mode of metastasis, but hematogenous spread to lung, liver, and bone occurs commonly. Amyloid deposits are seen in 85% to 90% of these tumors and are pathognomonic. The mean mortality rate is approximately 50%.

Histology

The tumor is usually infiltrative and grows in nests. Amyloid may be present in the stroma.

ANAPLASTIC CARCINOMA

Presentation

The usual presentation is is that of a rapidly enlarging neck mass.

Pathophysiology

Anaplastic carcinoma accounts for 10% of all thyroid cancers. It is more commonly seen in women over 50 years of age. The association between this tumor and preexisting goiter accounts for the increased prevalence of anaplastic tumors in areas where goiter is endemic. The current theory is that this tumor evolves from a previously well-differentiated cancer. The tumor grows rapidly, with aggressive local invasion. More than 50% of patients have disease beyond the neck at the time of presentation. The end result is generally dysphagia, airway obstruction, and exsanguination. Most patients die within 1 year of diagnosis.

Histology

Histologically, the tumor is divided into giant cell, spindle cell, and small cell types. It is now felt that many tumors previously identified as small-cell tumors are in fact lymphomas.

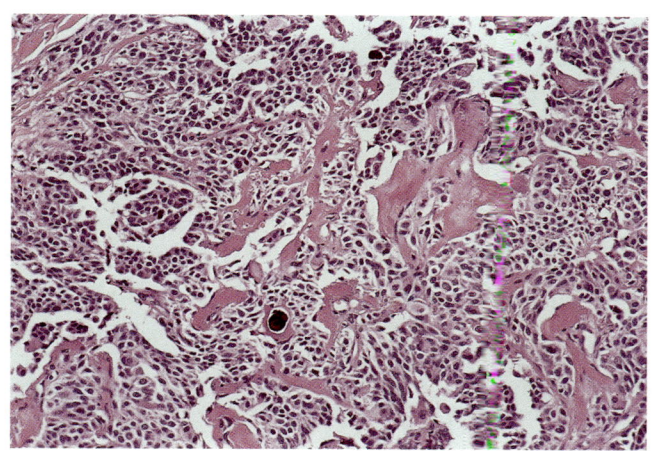

FIG. 2-17. Medullary carcinoma of the thyroid gland, showing amyloid stroma.

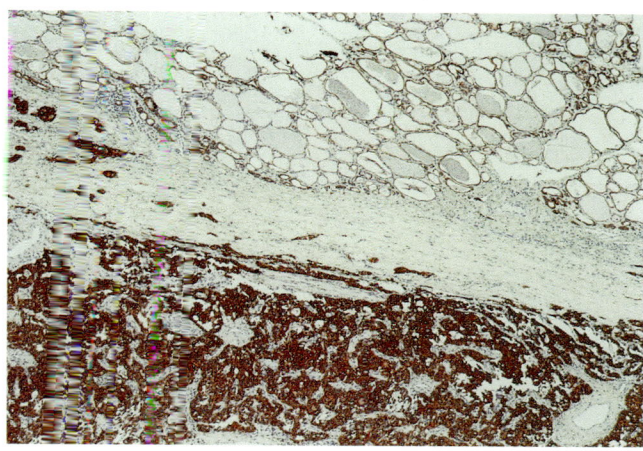

FIG. 2-18. Immunoreaction for calcitonin (*lower half*) in medullary carcinoma of the thyroid.

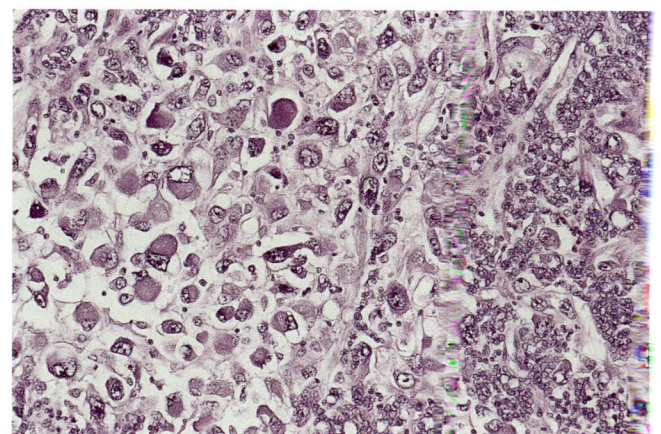
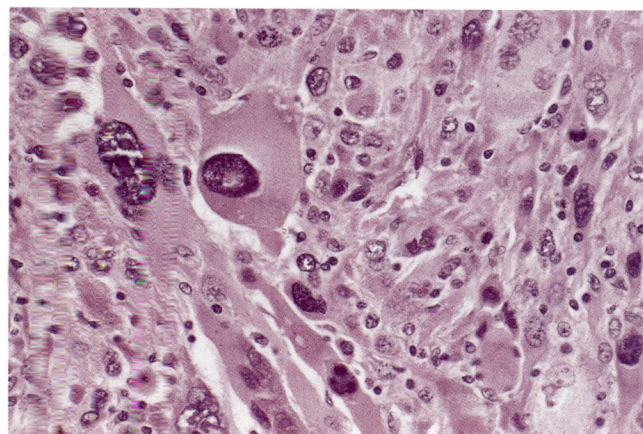

FIG. 2-19. A,B: Anaplastic (high-grade) carcinoma of the thyroid gland.

3

Parathyroid Gland

HYPERPARATHYROIDISM

Presentation

The diagnosis of hyperparathyroidism was uncommon until the 1960s and 1970s, when multichannel chemical analyzers were developed and first used to screen serum calcium levels during routine hospital admissions.

Pathophysiology

Hyperparathyroidism may be caused by either hyperplasia of the glands or an adenoma of a single gland.

Histology

Hyperplasia is characterized by an increased cellularity of all the glands and a decreased amount of fat within the glands.

A parathyroid adenoma may be difficult to distinguish from hyperplasia unless a rim of normal parathyroid tissue is present at the periphery of the adenoma. More commonly, a biopsy specimen is taken from a second, normal parathyroid gland and examined for comparison.

PARATHYROID CARCINOMA

Presentation

One should suspect carcinoma when the serum calcium level is exceptionally high or when, during surgery, a dense fibrous reaction is noted around the gland, causing it to adhere to surrounding structures.

Pathophysiology

Parathyroid carcinoma is extremely uncommon, comprising only 0.5% to 4% of all cases of primary hyperparathyroidism.

Histology

Histologically, one sees cytoplasmic and nuclear atypia and fibrosis separating neoplastic clusters.

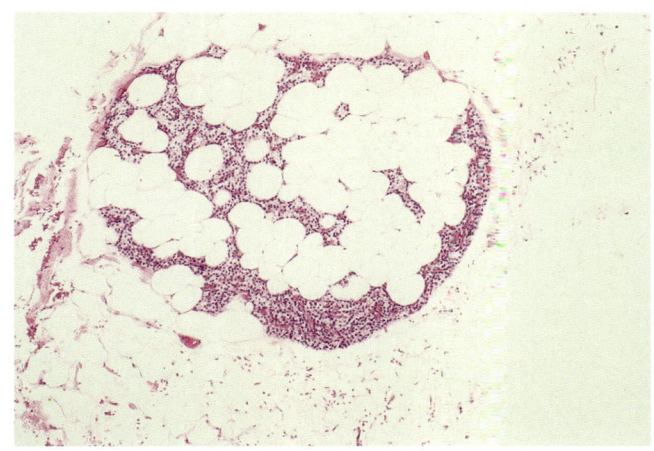

FIG. 3-1. Normal parathyroid.

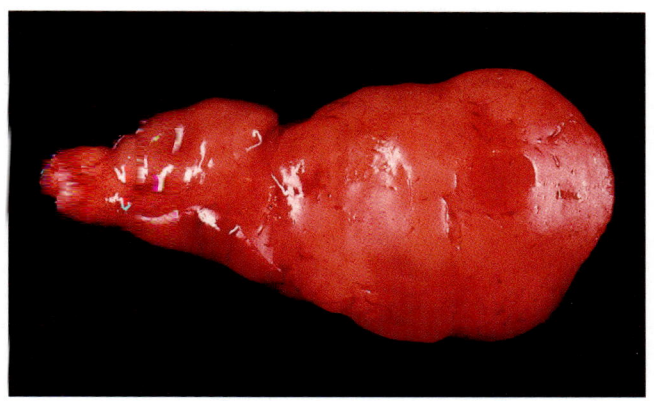

FIG. 3-2. Parathyroid gland adenoma.

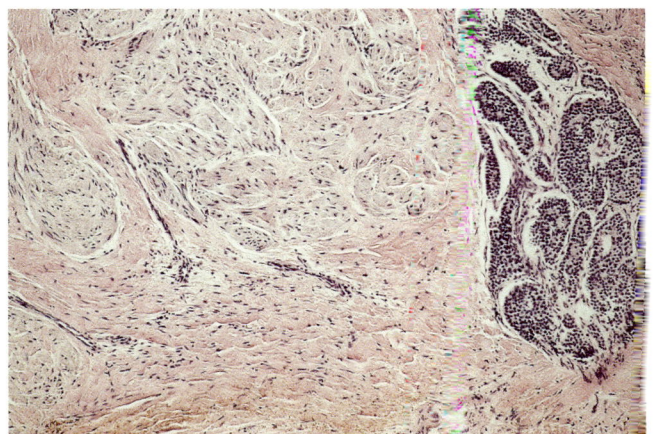

FIG. 3-3. Parathyroid carcinoma with extensive fibrosis.

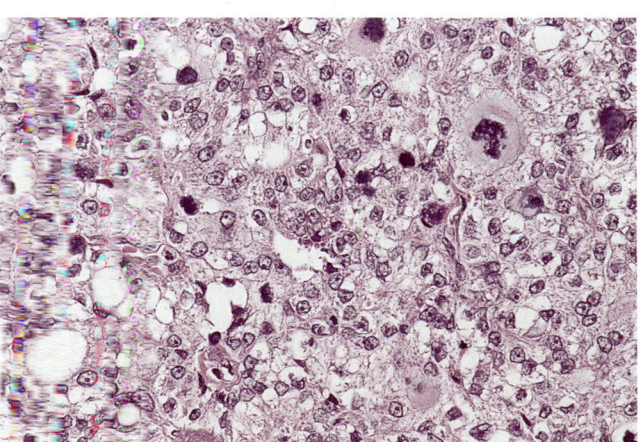

FIG. 3-4. Marked pleomorphism in a parathyroid gland carcinoma.

4
Ear

CERUMINOMA

Presentation

The usual presenting symptom is obstruction of the ear canal. Pain is uncommon unless there is associated inflammation.

Pathophysiology

Ceruminoma or apocrine adenoma is a benign tumor showing apocrine secretory differentiation. There are also malignant forms—ceruminous gland adenocarcinoma or apocrine carcinoma and adenoid cystic carcinoma.

Histology

The tumor is well demarcated, showing a glandular proliferation. Growth patterns include solid, cystic, and papillary. The glands are composed of two cell layers; the inner or luminal layer is cuboidal, and the outer is spindle-shaped.

CHOLESTEATOMA

Presentation

Clinically, cholesteatomas may be congenital, primary acquired, or secondary acquired. Virtually by definition, the first can be diagnosed only as a cholesteatomatous mass behind an intact eardrum. Primary acquired cholesteatoma is manifested by the classic posterior superior quadrant retraction pocket of the tympanic membrane. Secondary acquired cholesteatoma is believed to develop through a perforation in the tympanic membrane. Primary acquired cholesteatoma is by far the most common type.

Pathphysiology

In any case, the symptoms are a consequence of slow expansion of the choleasteatomatous mass, which causes bone erosion. This is felt to occur by several mechanisms. The first and most important probably involves an inflammatory response at the leading edge of the cholesteatoma, which causes the neighboring bone to dissolve, allowing the cholesteatoma to grow.

Histology

Histologically, a cholesteatoma is composed of keratinizing squamous epithelium with subepithelial fibroconnective tissue. It is generally associated with acute and chronic inflammation.

CHOLESTEROL GRANULOMA

Presentation

On otoscopy, one sees a blue-tinged mass behind an intact eardrum.

Pathophysiology

Cholesterol granuloma occurs as a result of a foreign body reaction to cholesterol crystals within the middle ear, generally felt to be secondary to a prior episode of hemorrhage.

Histology

Histologically, one sees an inflammatory response with scattered, slitlike spaces of cholesterol.

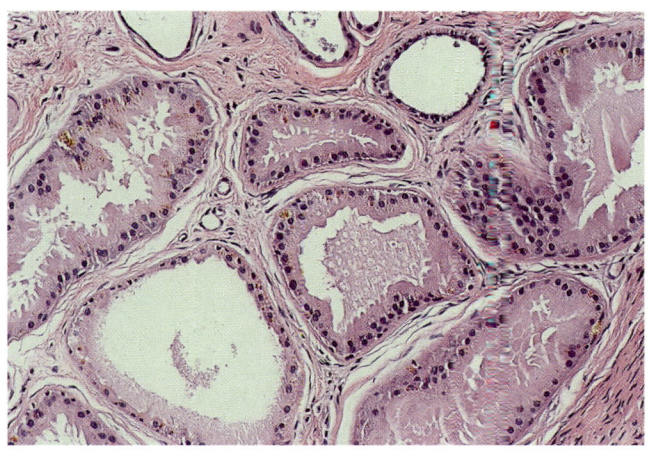

FIG. 4-1. Normal ceruminous gland of the lateral two-thirds of the external auditory canal.

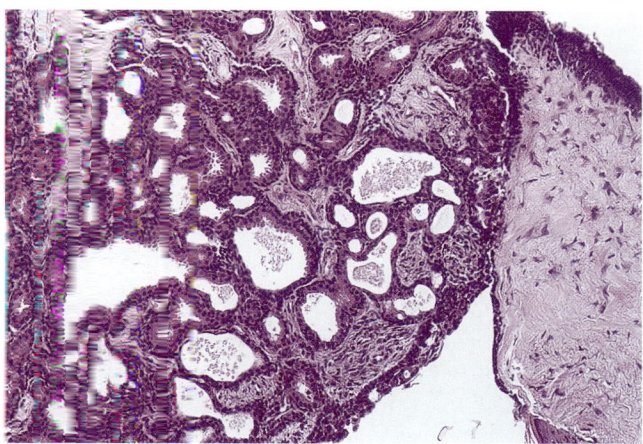

FIG. 4-2. Ceruminoma, a low-grade neoplasm.

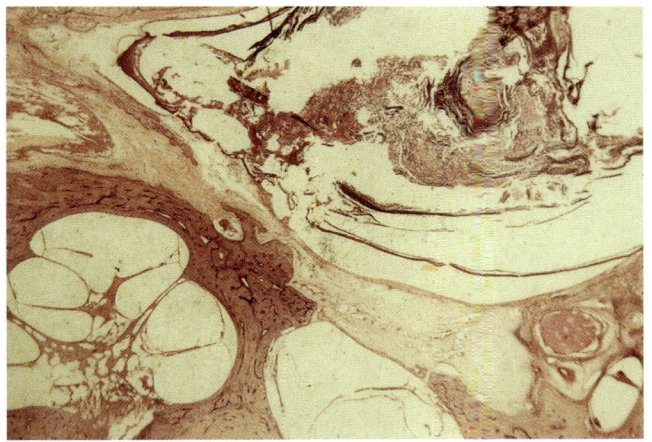

FIG. 4-3. Cholesteatoma showing keratinizing squamous epithelium with subepithelial fibroconnective tissue.

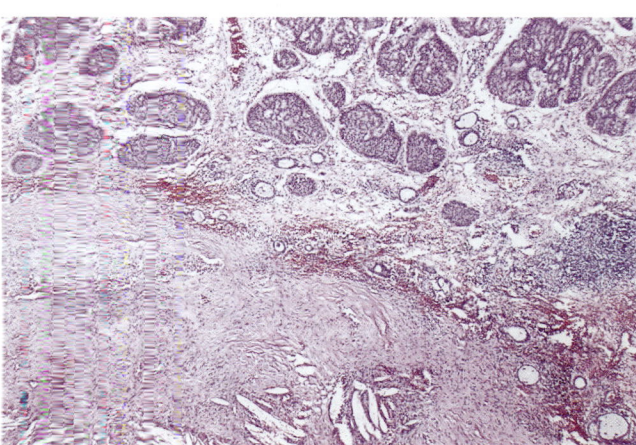

FIG. 4-4. Adenomatous tumor of the middle ear accompanied by a cholesterol granuloma.

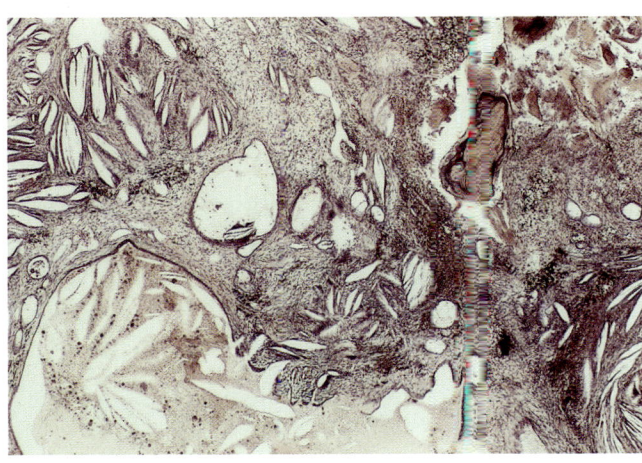

FIG. 4-5. Cholesterol granuloma showing inflammatory response with scattered slit-like spaces of cholesterol.

MALIGNANT EXTERNAL OTITIS (NECROTIZING EXTERNAL OTITIS)

Presentation

This potentially fatal infection of the external auditory canal is caused by *Pseudomonas aeruginosa*. It tends to occur in immunocompromised persons, particularly those with uncontrolled diabetes mellitus.

Pathophysiology

The disease tends to spread through the tympanomastoid suture and then along the base of the skull, potentially affecting a number of cranial nerves. A nearly pathognomonic physical sign is the presence of granulation tissue at the tympanomastoid suture in association with external otitis.

Histology

Histologically, there is granulation tissue with acute and chronic inflammation and necrosis.

ACUTE OTITIS MEDIA

Presentation

The most common symptoms are otalgia and hearing loss, and the tympanic membrane will be red and bulging.

Pathophysiology

Acute otitis media is an acute inflammatory infection of the middle ear, usually caused by *Streptococcus pneumoniae* or *Haemophilus influenzae*. It is a common disease in children and much less common in adults.

Histology

Histologically, the tissues show an acute inflammatory infection.

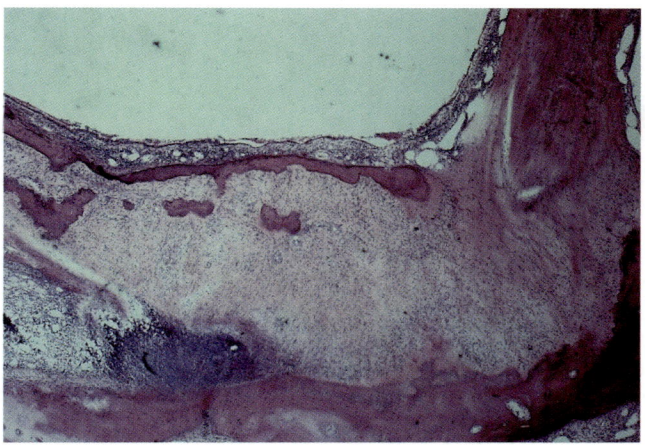

FIG. 4-6. Malignant external otitis showing granulation tissue with acute and chronic inflammation and necrosis.

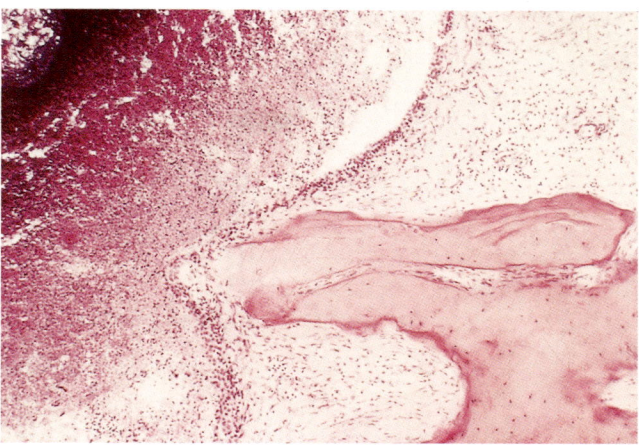

FIG. 4-7. Acute otitis media showing acute inflammatory response.

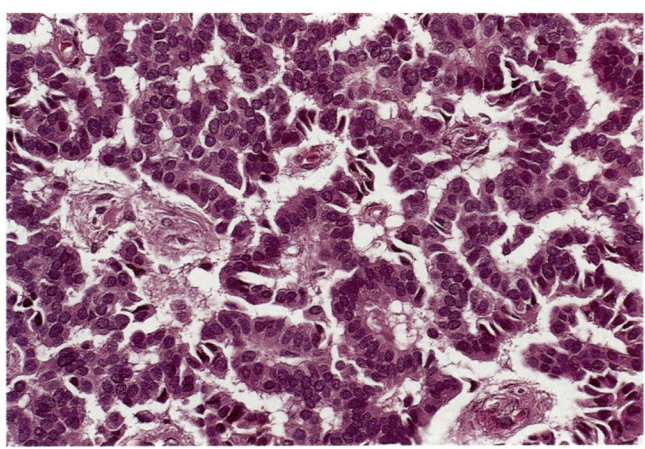

FIG. 4-8. Adenomatous tumor of the middle ear manifesting a carcinoid pattern of cytoarchitecture.

EOSINOPHILIC GRANULOMA

Presentation

This disease of cryptogenic etiology is one of a group of lesions referred to collectively as histiocytosis X or Langerhans cell histiocytosis; the group also comprises Letterer-Siwe syndrome and Hand-Schüller-Christian disease. Eosinophilic granuloma occurs more frequently in male patients, most often in the second and third decades of life. The most commonly affected sites are the middle ear and temporal bone.

Pathophysiology

Symptoms usually include otorrhea, otitis media, bone pain, and loss of hearing.

Histology

Histologically, there is a proliferation of histiocytic cells in clusters, nests, or sheets. The cells have round, vesicular nuclei with a lobulated or indented nuclear membrane and eosinophilic cytoplasm. There is in addition an admixture of other inflammatory cells, predominantly eosinophils. Multinucleated giant cells may also be present. The histiocytes are S100-positive.

ENDOLYMPHATIC SAC TUMORS

Presentation

Endolymphatic sac tumors are rare neuroectodermal "neoplasms" in the petrous bone. They seem to originate from inner ear structures and may occur sporadically or in von Hippel-Lindau disease. The most common symptoms are sensorineural deafness and tinnitus, with a smaller number of patients experiencing imbalance.

Pathophysiology

The tumors are slowly enlarging masses within the petrous bone, generally reddish or bluish in color and hypervascular in appearance. They are soft and tend to bleed when manipulated.

Histology

Histologically, there are two common patterns. The first pattern consists of colloid-filled cysts with a sparse stroma; the colloid stains strongly with periodic acid–Schiff but is negative for mucicarmine. The second growth pattern is papillary and solid with prominent clear cells. The papillary structures are abundant, and the stroma is characterized by numerous capillaries.

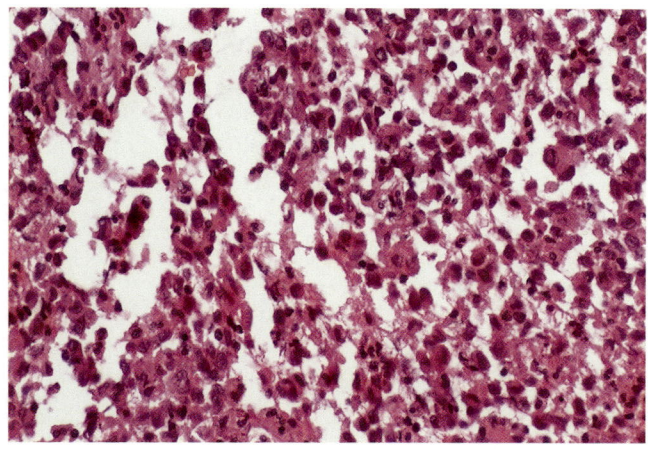

FIG. 4-9. Photomicrograph of eosinophilic granuloma showing eosinophilic infiltrate.

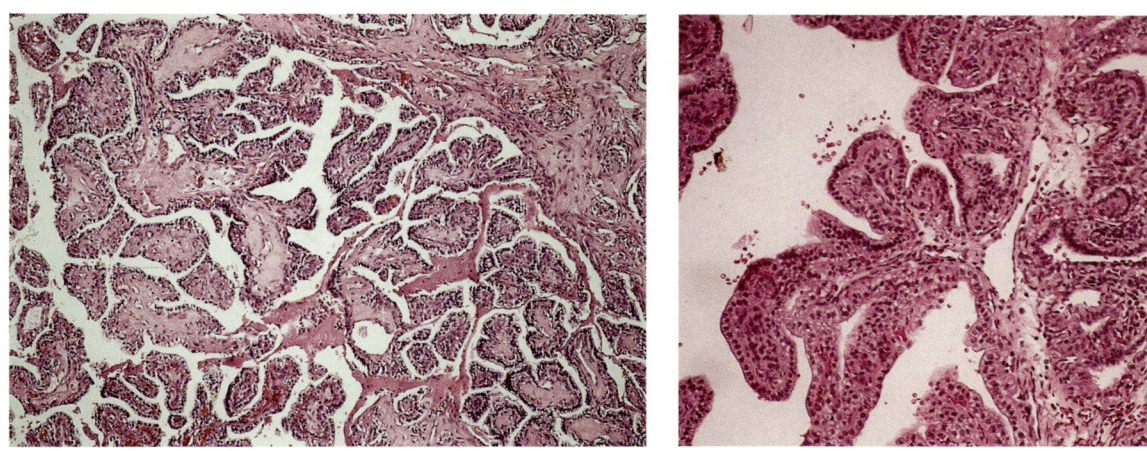

FIG. 4-10. A,B: Papillary endolymphatic sac tumor.

5
Larynx

VOCAL FOLD NODULES

Presentation

The patient will present with hoarseness, usually painless.

Pathophysiology

Vocal fold nodules may occur in all age groups and are thought to be caused by vocal abuse. They usually occur bilaterally at the juncture of the anterior and middle two-thirds of the true vocal fold.

Histology

The histology can be quite varied depending on the severity of the nodules and how long they have been present, but deposition of fibrous tissue is always present in the submucosa.

CONTACT GRANULOMAS AND ULCERS

Presentation

The patient usually presents with hoarseness or pain on vocalization. Large lesions may obstruct the airway. There is usually a history of trauma, and acid reflux nearly always plays a role.

Pathophysiology

Contact granulomas and ulcers of the larynx typically develop in the posterior aspect of the vocal fold, generally in the area of the vocal process. Men are more often affected than women. These lesions occur in patients of a wide age range, although generally in adults. The probable etiologic factors are numerous, but vocal abuse and acid reflux laryngitis and pharyngitis are frequently involved. The lesions may also be secondary to trauma, such as endotracheal intubation. They typically appear either unilaterally or bilaterally as nodular but focally ulcerated masses in the area of the vocal process of the vocal fold.

Histology

Histologically, these lesions show fibrinoid necrosis and granulation tissue with both acute and chronic inflammation, the ratio depending on the age of the lesion.

SQUAMOUS PAPILLOMA

Presentation

Patients usually present with painless hoarseness. Airway compromise will occur as the disease progresses.

Pathophysiology

Squamous papillomas, the most common benign laryngeal tumors in children, are areas of proliferation of stratified squamous epithelium. Malignant transformation is rare. They are thought to be caused by the human papillomavirus, and a history of genital papillomas is present in 29% of mothers of affected children. These lesions tend to be multiple in location and unremitting in course. They may also occur in adults, although less commonly, and tend to follow the same course.

Histology

Histologically, one sees benign proliferation of stratified squamous epithelium forming papillary fronds with a fibrovascular core.

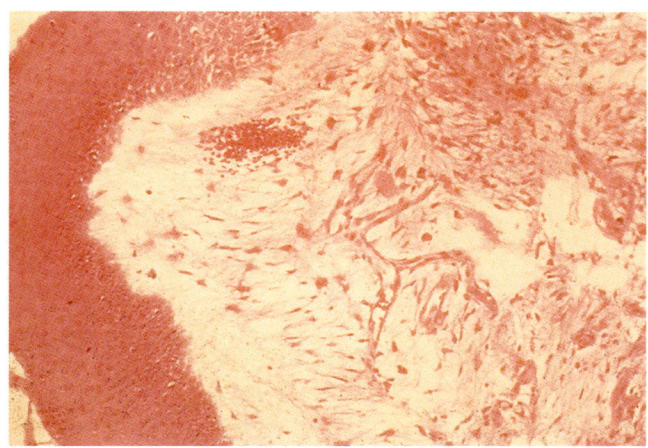
FIG. 5-1. Vocal fold nodules.

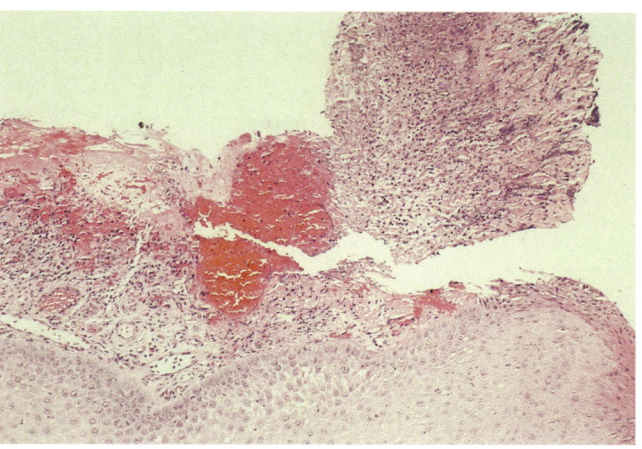
FIG. 5-2. Contact granuloma.

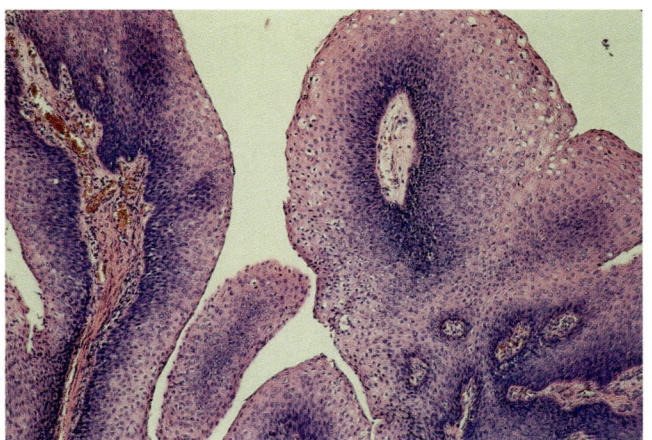
FIG. 5-3. Laryngeal papillomas. Note vascular cores and the minimal surface keratin.

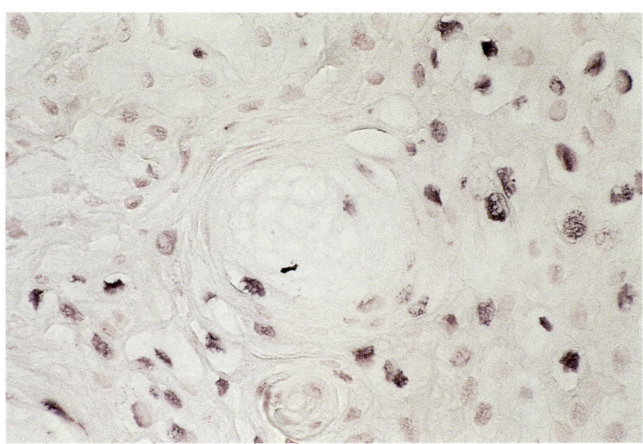
FIG. 5-4. Positive nuclear immunostaining for human papillomavirus DNA in a papilloma of the larynx.

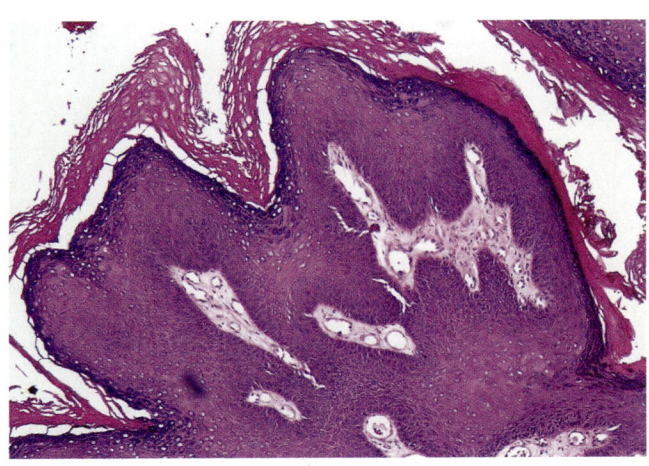
FIG. 5-5. Keratinizing papilloma in oral cavity.

6
Sinonasal

NASAL POLYPS

Presentation

The cause of nasal polyps is unknown, but approximately 50% of these patients will have a skin test result that is positive for environmental allergens. The polyp itself is made up of nasal mucous membrane having large amounts of edematous fluid, sparse fibrous cells, and few mucous glands.

Pathophysiology

Polyps may be single but usually are multiple or bilateral. They cause a constant mucopurulent rhinorrhea and progressive nasal obstruction.

Histology

The surface epithelium usually shows squamous metaplasia, whereas the supporting tissues contain lymphocytes, plasma cells, eosinophils, and mast cells. In addition, levels of IgA, IgE, IgG, and IgM are elevated within the tissues. On the histologic examination, the surface epithelium is intact, and the stroma shows marked edema with an inflammatory infiltrate.

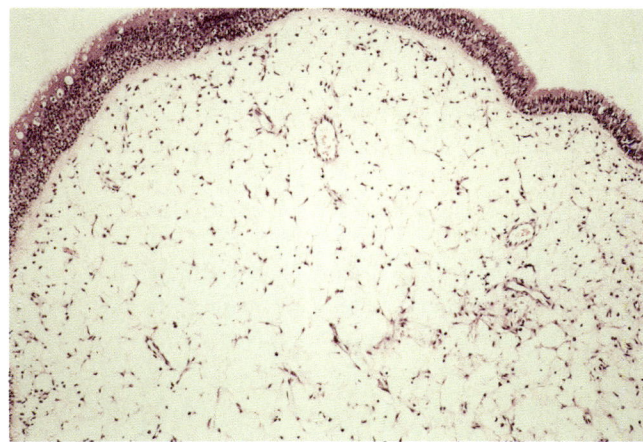

FIG. 6-1. Nasal polyp.

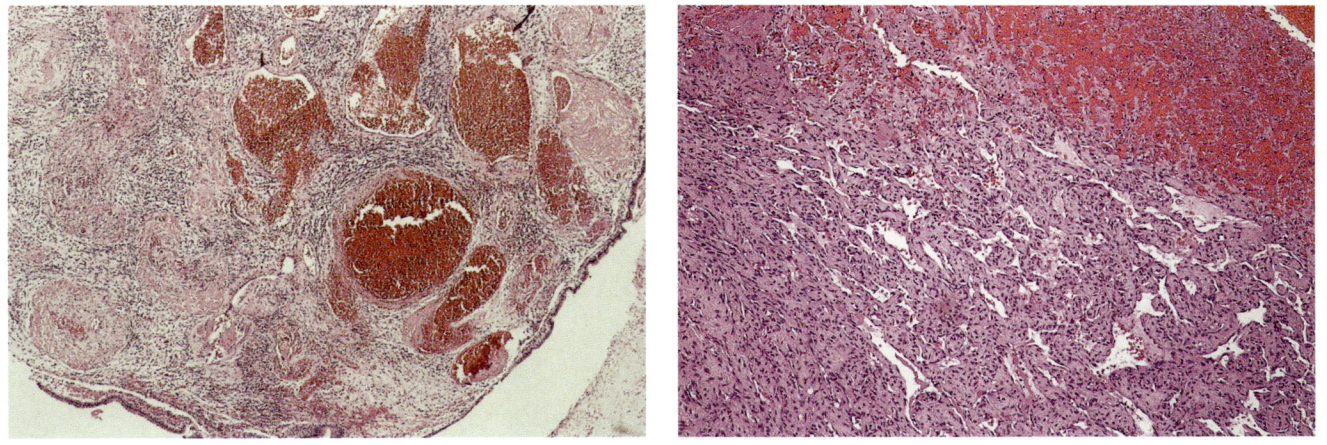

FIG. 6-2. A,B: Angiomatous nasal polyp. The vascular formation is unlike that of a hemangioma or angiofibroma and is characterized by vascular compromise, infarct, and neovascularization.

ALLERGIC FUNGAL SINUSITIS

Presentation

The majority of patients with allergic fungal sinusitis present with a long history of progressive nasal airway obstruction, either unilateral or bilateral.

Pathophysiology

The exact pathophysiology of this disease is uncertain, but it is clear that an exuberant "allergic" reaction to the presence of fungus within the sinus or sinuses involved is occurring. There is no fungal invasion of the mucosa, but the mucosa shows marked edema with a lush eosinophilic infiltration.

Histology

The fungal elements can be found only in the allergic mucin, which contains aggregates of eosinophils and Charcot-Leyden crystals. The mucosa itself is markedly edematous with eosinophilic infiltrate.

MUCORMYCOSIS

Presentation

Mucormycosis is generally seen in patients with an underlying immunosuppressive disease, typically diabetic ketoacidosis or AIDS. The causative organisms are species of *Absidia*, *Mucor*, and *Rhizopus*. The disease is usually characterized by acute rhinosinusitis with facial cellulitis and gangrenous mucosal changes. Nasal examination reveals brick red or black tissue that is anesthetic and does not bleed.

Pathophysiology

The organism invades along vascular channels, causing a vascular necrosis as it spreads. It may in certain situations rapidly spread intracranially and cause blindness, ophthalmoplegia, and cavernous sinus thrombosis.

Histology

There is tissue necrosis and vascular invasion by broad, nonseptate hyphae.

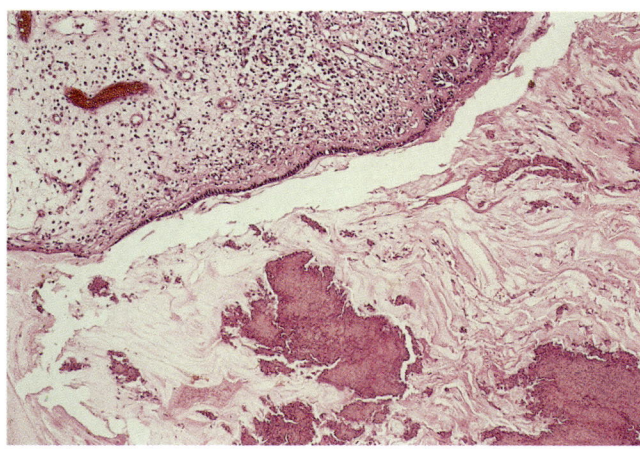

FIG. 6-3. Allergic fungal sinusitis. The allergic mucin lies below and does not invade the underlying sinus tissue.

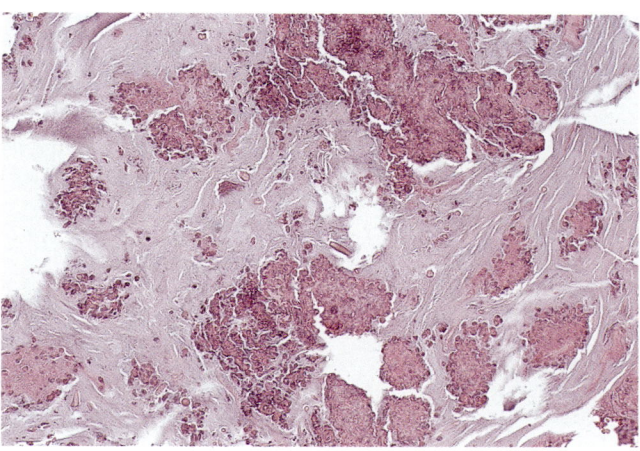

FIG. 6-4. Allergic fungal sinusitis. The allergic mucin contains numerous aggregates of eosinophils, Charcot-Leyden crystals, and cellular debris.

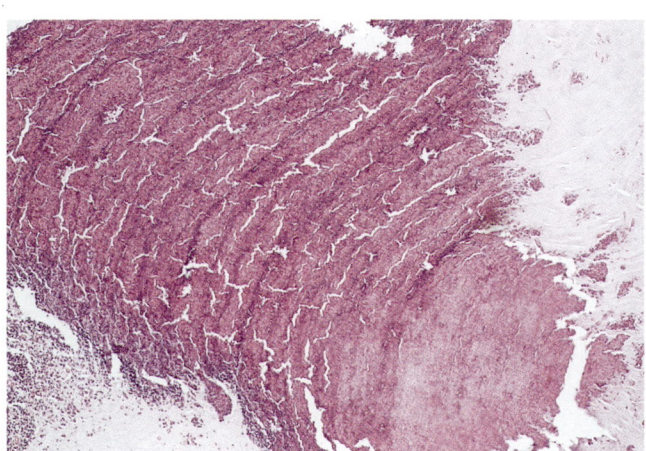

FIG. 6-5. Typical laminated aggregate of cellular debris, eosinophils, and crystals in allergic fungal sinusitis.

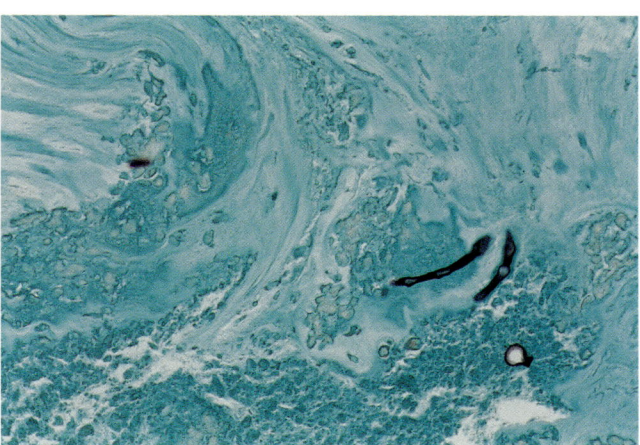

FIG. 6-6. Allergic fungal sinusitis with *Bipolaris* fungal hyphae in mucin.

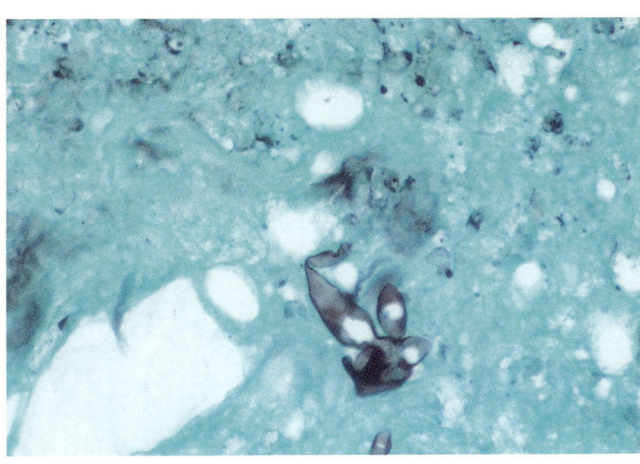

FIG. 6-7. Mucormycosis in the sinus of a immunocompromised patient.

MYOSPHERULOSIS

Presentation

Myospherulosis generally occurs after an operative procedure in which ointment-impregnated gauze is used within the nasal cavity. The late presentation is a chronic, unremitting inflammatory response in a localized area.

Pathophysiology

This disease results when petroleum-based ointment penetrates underneath the mucosa, producing an intense inflammatory response.

Histology

One sees a submucosal intensive inflammatory reaction and the shadow of the petroleum ointment and pseudofungal aggregates of erythrocytes.

WEGENER'S GRANULOMATOSIS

Presentation

There is a slight male predominance, and the peak incidence is in the fourth to fifth decades. Wegener's granulomatosis involves the nose and paranasal sinuses in 90% of patients. In 60% of cases, the ears are also affected.

Pathophysiology

An immune-based disease, Wegener's granulomatosis affects many organ systems, but preferentially the upper and lower respiratory tracts and kidneys.

Histology

Histologically, the disease is characterized by a necrotizing granulomatous vasculitis involving small and medium-sized arteries with an inflammatory infiltrate.

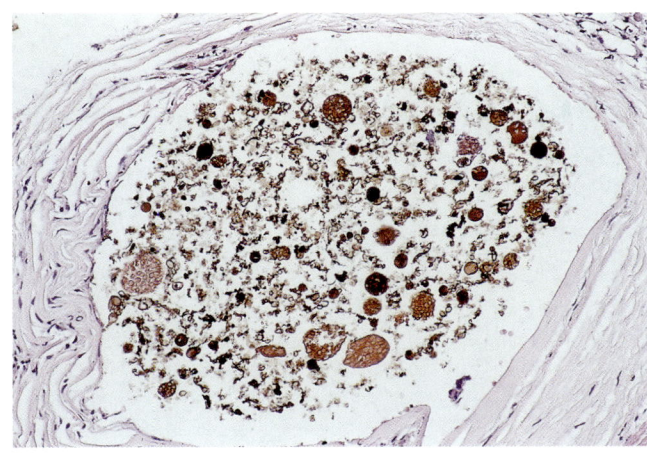

FIG. 6-8. Myospherulosis of the nasal cavity.

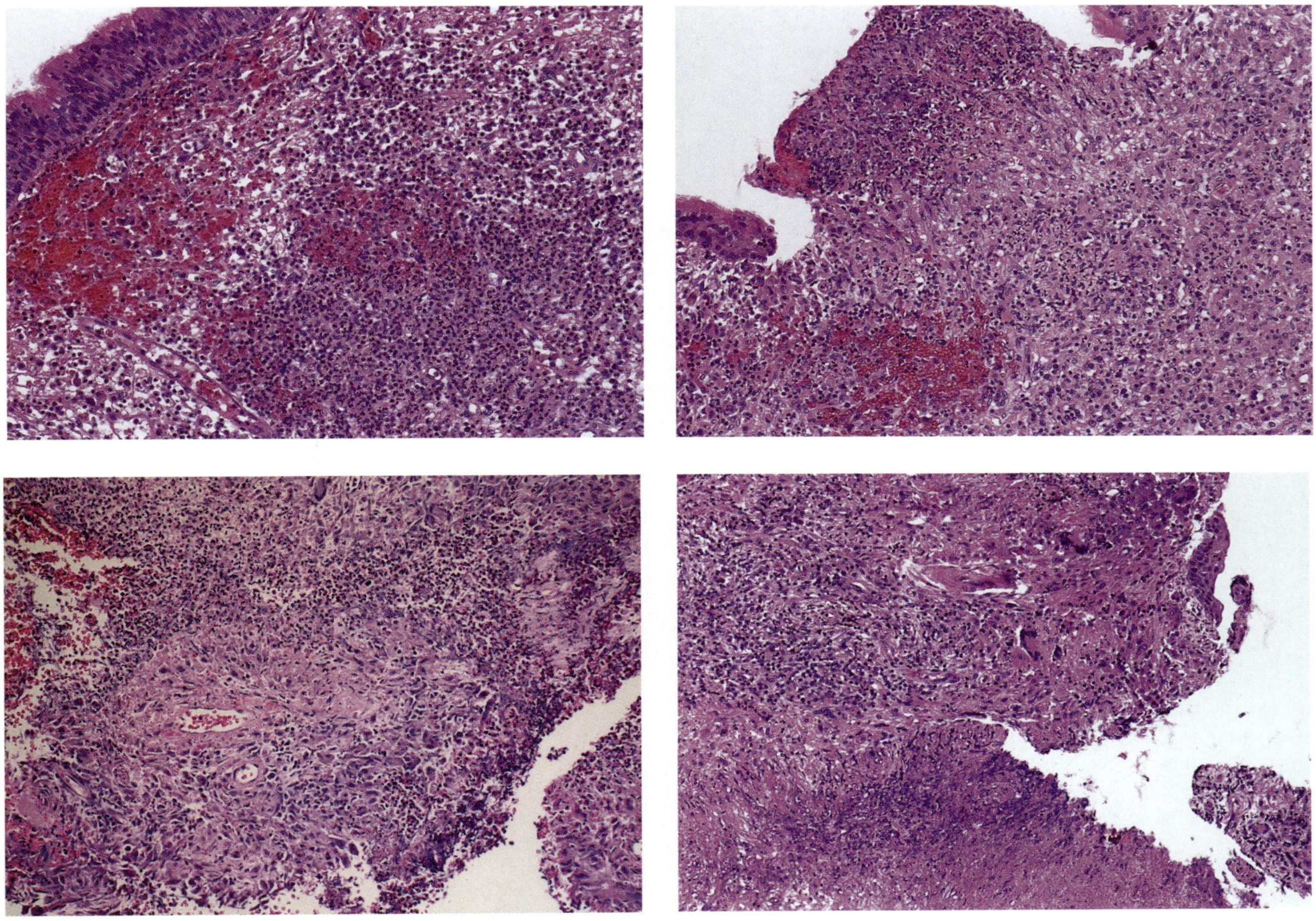

FIG. 6-9. A–D: Wegener's granulomatosis of the nasal cavity, showing the sequence from vasculitis and microabscess in **A** to mucosal ulcer in **B** and more extensive necrosis in **C** and **D**.

INVERTED PAPILLOMA

Presentation

Inverted papilloma is a benign tumor of the lateral nasal wall or sinus. The patient usually presents with nasal obstruction.

Pathophysiology

A relationship of the tumor to squamous cell carcinoma is variously reported in the literature as being between 8% and 50%; a more reasonable estimate is 13%. The average age range of patients is from 40 to 70 years, with a slight male predominance.

Histology

Histologically, the lesions show an ingrowing pattern of thickened, pseudostratified schneiderian epithelium, which inverts into the stoma. The counterpart on the septum is fungiform in structure and rarely related to a carcinoma.

FUNGIFORM PAPILLOMA

Presentation

The patient usually presents with unilateral nasal obstruction, occasionally with epistaxis.

Pathophysiology

This papilloma is usually a well-demarcated lesion on the septum that can generally be easily excised.

Histology

Histologically, the lesion consists of benign squamous epithelium forming papillary fronds with a fibrous core.

ANGIOFIBROMA

Presentation

Angiofibroma is an uncommon, histologically benign tumor that occurs almost exclusively in male adolescents. The most common initial symptom is epistaxis unrelated to trauma, although nasal obstruction will occur as the tumor grows.

Pathophysiology

The tumor is locally invasive and may penetrate the nasal cavity, orbit, and intracranial cavity.

Histology

Histologically, the tumor is unencapsulated and shows an admixture of large vascular spaces lying in a fibrous stroma. Vascular spaces are thin-walled and lack a muscular layer.

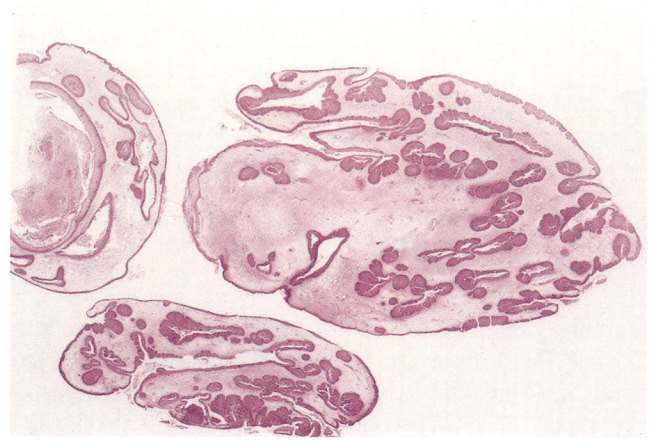

FIG. 6-10. Schneiderian papilloma of the lateral nasal wall.

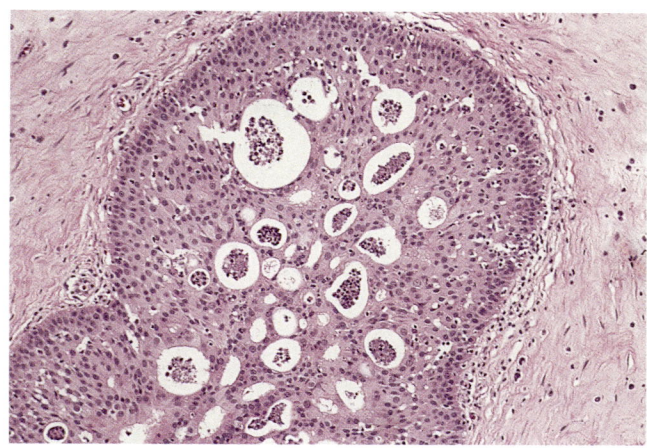

FIG. 6-11. Lateral wall schneiderian papilloma.

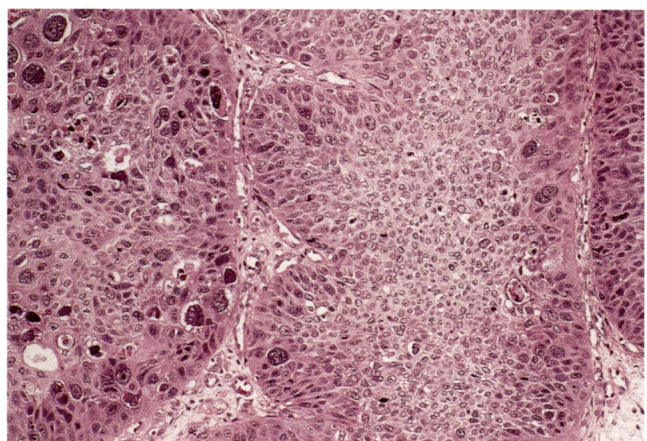

FIG. 6-12. Carcinoma arising in schneiderian papilloma of the lateral wall.

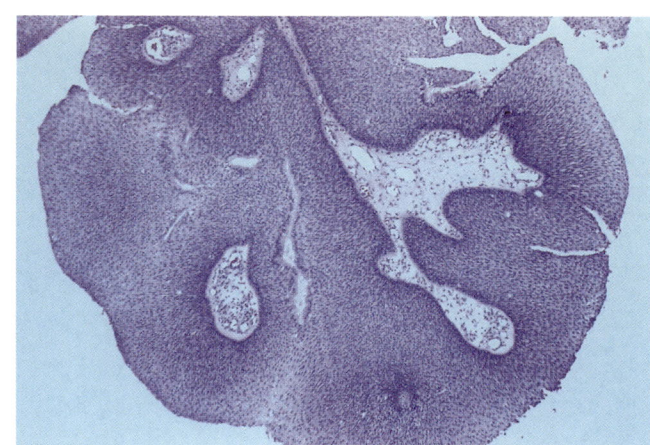

FIG. 6-13. Septal (fungiform) schneiderian papilloma. These papillomas may have an inverting component, but the exophytic character dominates.

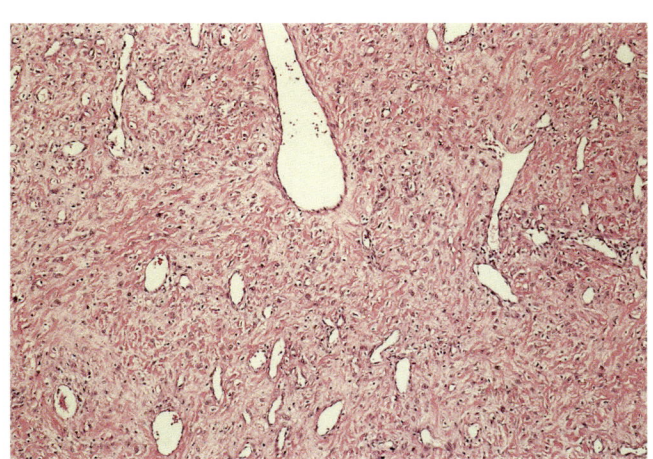
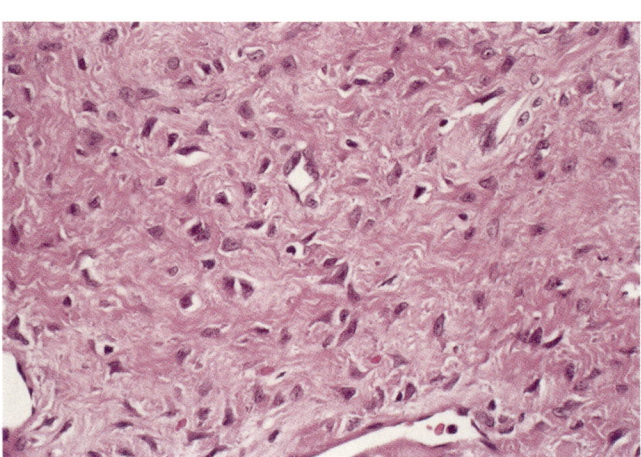

FIG. 6-14. Angiofibroma of the postnasal space.

ADENOCARCINOMAS

Presentation

Adenocarcinomas occur most commonly in the sinonasal tract and present with nasal obstruction. In other locations, they are generally asymptomatic masses at first; symptoms appear later and are site-dependent. Epidemiologically, exposure to wood dust is a major factor in some adenocarcinomas.

Pathophysiology

Adenocarcinomas are the second most common malignant tumors of the sinonasal tract. They show a glandular formation and are of surface or seromucous epithelial origin. They tend to involve the ethmoid sinus most commonly. A particularly distinctive type of sinonasal adenocarcinoma is the "enteric" adenocarcinoma, in which cytologic findings are analogous to those in carcinomas of the gastrointestinal tract.

Histology

Surface adenocarcinoma are of the "conventional" adenocarcinoma type. The seromucous glands give rise to adenoid cystic and low grade seromucous adenocarcinoma as the predominant types.

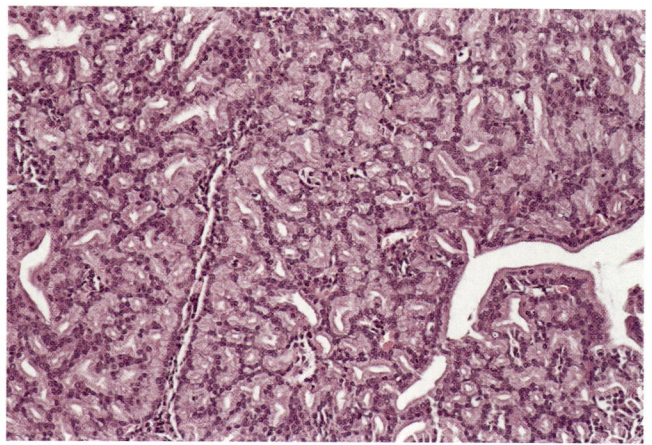

FIG. 6-15. Low-grade seromucous adenocarcinoma of the nasal cavity. Note the possible difficulty in differentiating this entity from hyperplasia of minor salivary glands.

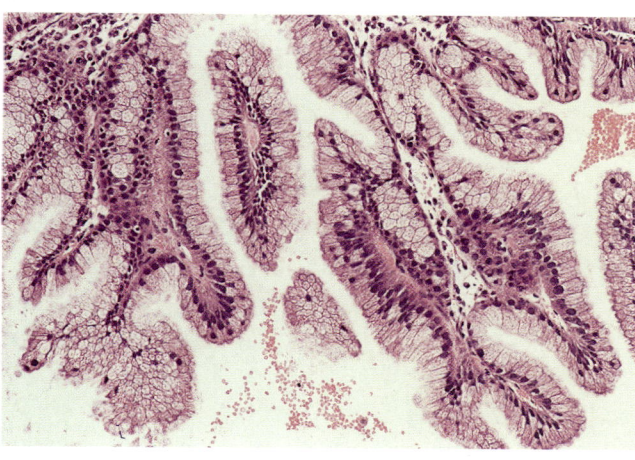

FIG. 6-16. Low-grade papillary surface-origin adenocarcinoma. Compare rather the banal appearance with the high-grade adenocarcinomas seen in Fig. 6-17.

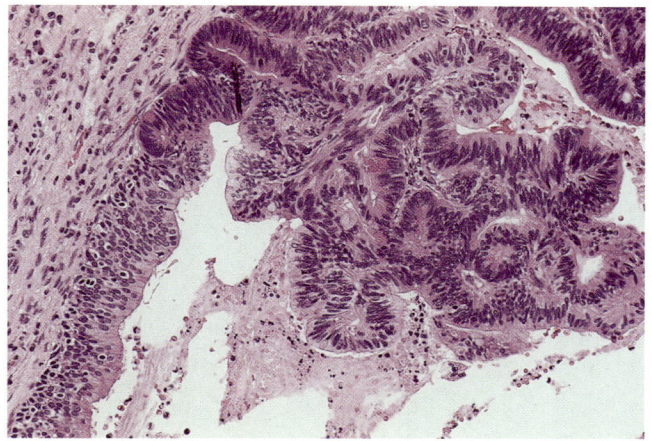

FIG. 6-17. High-grade paranasal sinus adenocarcinoma. Note the rather abrupt origin from the sinus mucosa.

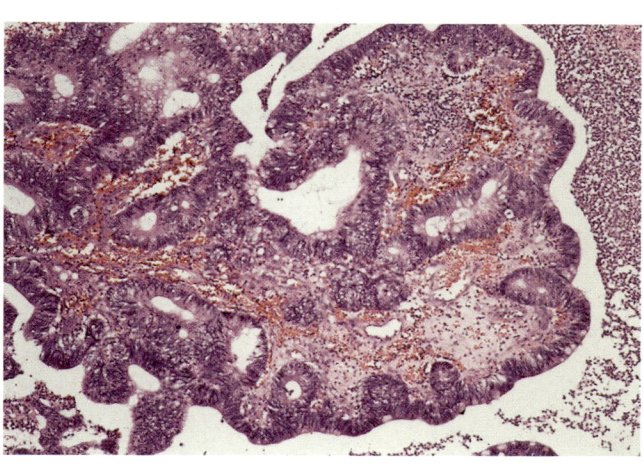

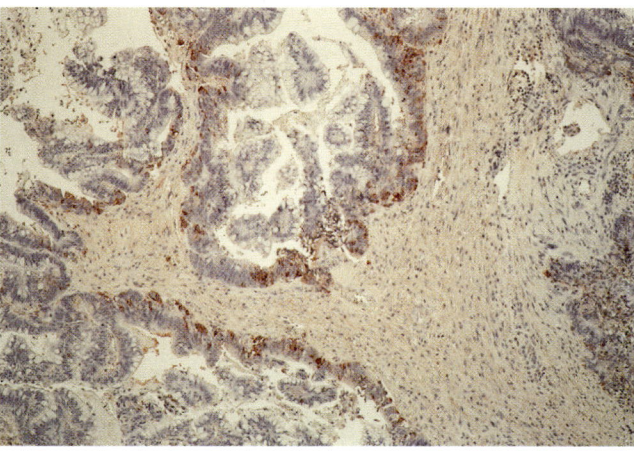

FIG. 6-19. "Enteric" type of adenocarcinoma stained to demonstrate serotonin in cells.

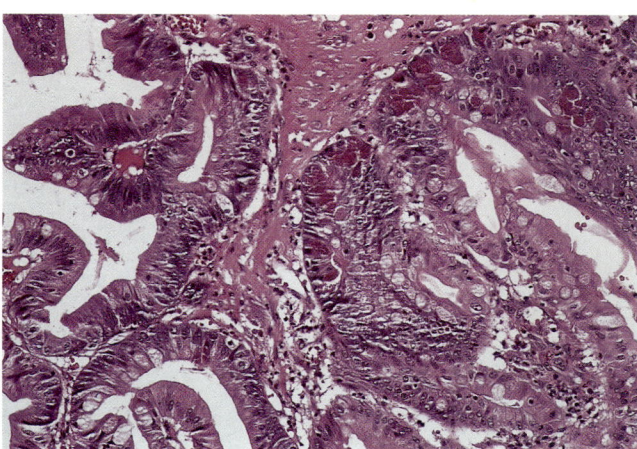

FIG. 6-18. A,B: "Enteric" type of high-grade adenocarcinoma of paranasal sinus. Note the Paneth's cell metaplasia in **B**.

OLFACTORY NEUROBLASTOMA

Presentation

Olfactory neuroblastoma generally presents as nasal obstruction, with or without epistaxis and with or without anosmia.

Pathophysiology

This tumor arises from the olfactory epithelium and thus tends to occur in the upper third of the nasal vault around the nasal septum and cribriform plate. It affects persons of a wide age range, but most patients are between the ages of 10 and 30.

Histology

There are four histologic grades for this tumor, with grade 1 being the most differentiated and grade 4 the least differentiated. Grade 1 tumors have a lobular architecture with little or no pleomorphism. Pleomorphism is significant in grade 2. Grade 3 may or may not be lobular, but pleomorphism is prominent. Pleomorphism is marked in grade 4. In the latter two grades, the neurofibrillary pattern is usually absent. The cells are usually cytokeratin-negative and chromogranin-positive, with positivity for S100 around peripheral lobular cells. Differential diagnosis includes neuroendocrine carcinoma and undifferentiated sinonasal carcinoma. Neuroendocrine carcinomas are more often keratin-positive and do not have a neurofibrillary matrix.

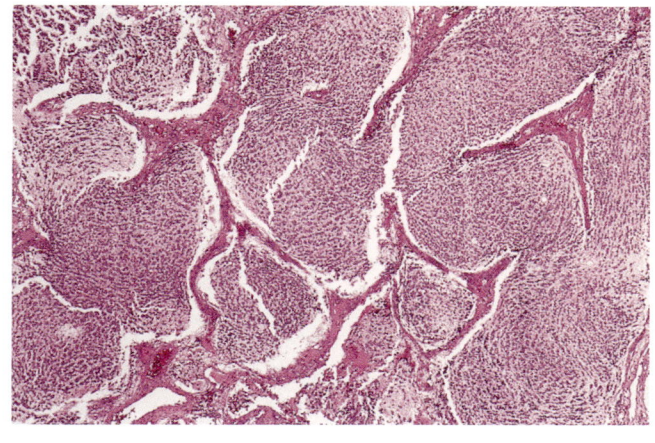
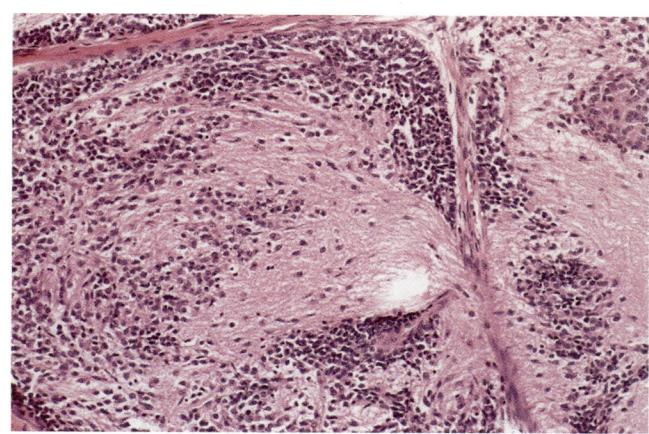
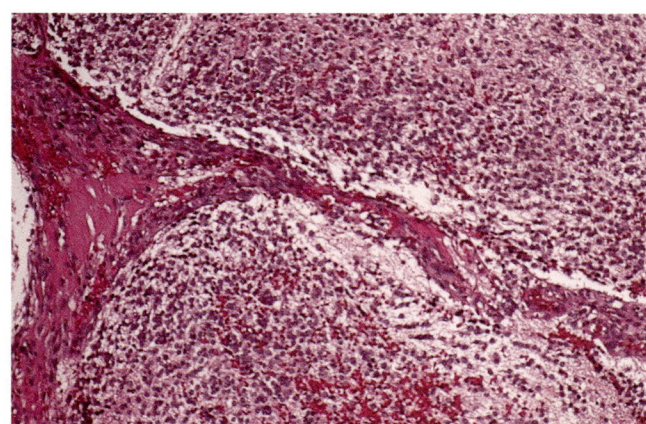

FIG. 6-20. A–C: Olfactory neuroblastoma. The small neurogenous cells and the neurofibrillary matrix make the diagnosis unequivocal.

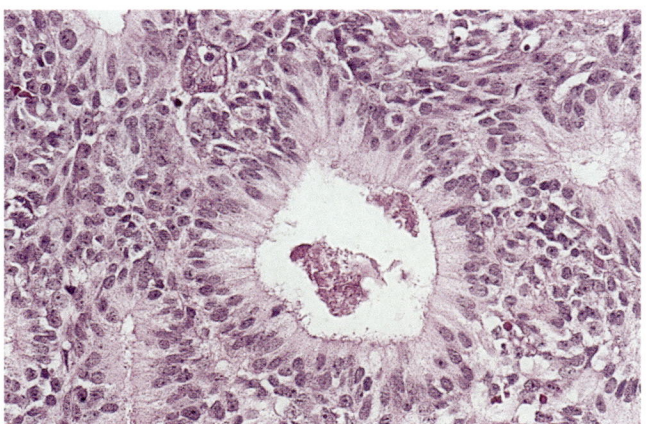

FIG. 6-21. Olfactory differentiation in this olfactory neuroblastoma is striking.

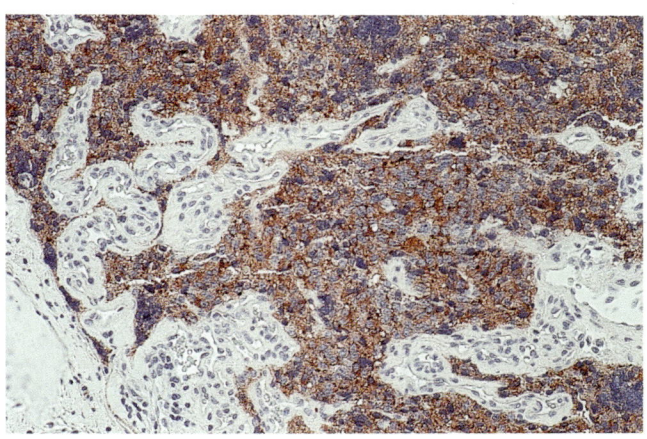

FIG. 6-22. Marked chromogranin immunoreactivity in an olfactory neuroblastoma.

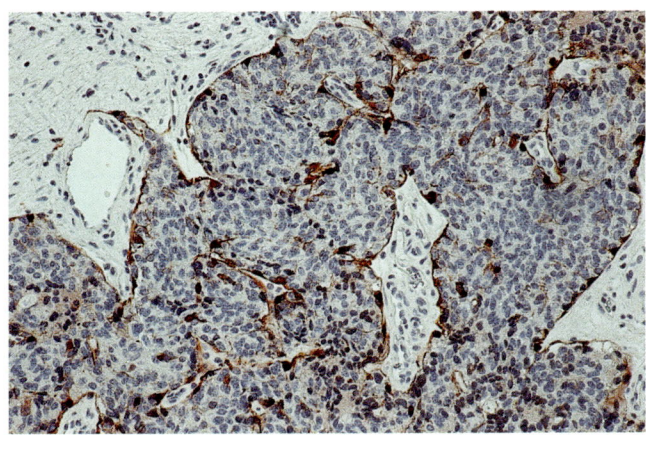

FIG. 6-23. Typical S100 protein reactivity in an olfactory neuroblastoma.

7

Skin and Fibrous Tissue

JUNCTIONAL NEVUS

Presentation

Junctional nevi generally appear in childhood.

Pathophysiology

These lesions are sharply circumscribed, hyperpigmented macules.

Histology

Melanocytes are seen at the epidermal-dermal junction.

COMPOUND NEVUS

Presentation

Compound nevi are papular.

Pathophysiology

Compound nevi tend to be lighter in color than junctional nevi.

Histology

In this case, the melanocytes are seen not only at the dermal-epidermal junction but also extending more deeply into the dermis.

INTRADERMAL NEVUS

Presentation

Intradermal nevus is the common nevus of older adults.

Pathophysiology

Intradermal nevi are typically dome-shaped, may be smooth or verrucous, and are generally flesh-colored. They may contain large terminal hairs.

Histology

Histologic examination shows the melanocytes to be situated primarily within the dermis.

ACTINIC KERATOSIS

Presentation

Actinic keratosis is probably the most sensitive indicator of lifetime sun exposure. These lesions generally present in areas of sun-damaged skin as rough spots that are more easily felt than visualized early on.

Pathophysiology

Over time, the keratotic scale thickens and acquires a yellow-brown color with or without surrounding erythema. If the nature of a lesion is in doubt, a biopsy should be performed.

Histology

These lesions are considered premalignant and show varying degrees of dysplasia. Often, parakeratosis and hyperkeratosis are present. Elastosis is also frequent.

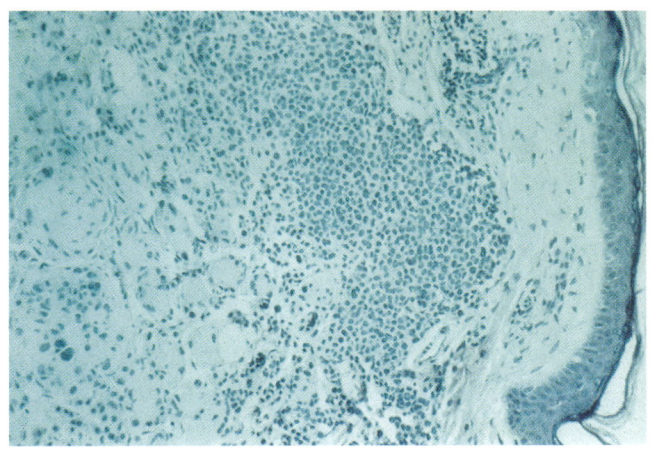

FIG. 7-1. Junctional nevus showing few melanocytes at the epidermal-dermal junction.

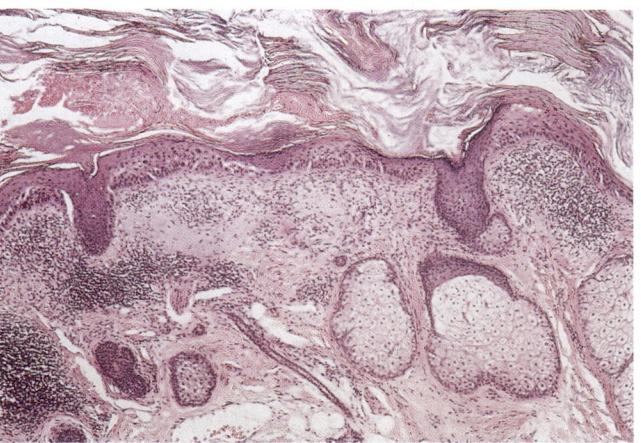

FIG. 7-2. Solar keratosis.

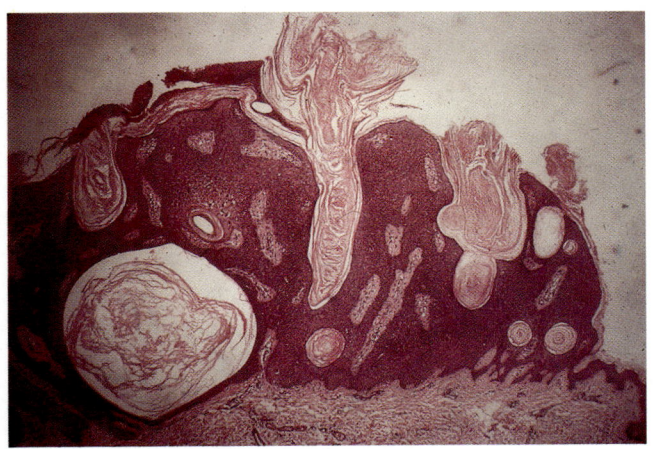

FIG. 7-3. Seborreic keratosis.

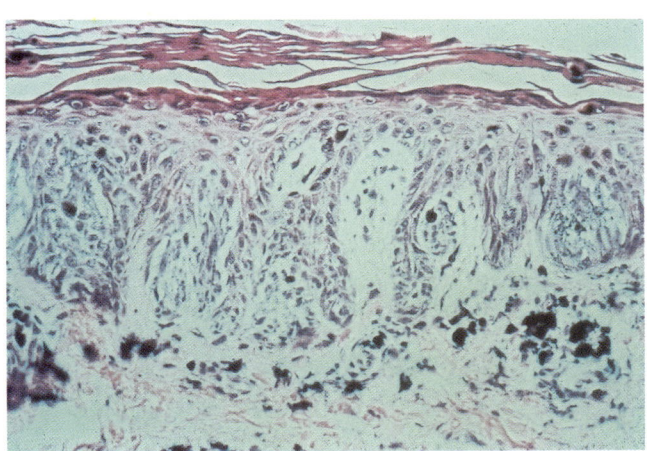

FIG. 7-4. Cutaneous melanoma.

SEBORRHEIC KERATOSIS

Presentation

Seborrheic keratoses are common skin lesions that generally appear after the age of 30 on hairy areas, particularly the trunk, the temple and surrounding areas, and the hands.

Pathophysiology

The lesions generally appear first as flesh-colored, slightly granular papules that grow in circumference, often with uneven pigmentation. The overlying surface is greasy and slightly verrucous.

Histology

Histologically, there is proliferation of basal cells within the epithelium.

FIBROUS TUMORS

Presentation

Fibrous lesions of the head and neck form a broad continuum ranging from keloids to fibrosarcomas. In between are a variety of diverse-appearing lesions. A broad term to denote the presence of such lesions is fibromatosis. These tumors almost always present as an enlarging mass, but their characteristics are otherwise widely divergent.

Pathophysiology

The pathophysiology of fibrous tumors is largely unknown or speculative.

Histology

Histologically, the lesions encompass a spectrum ranging from desmoid tumors to fibrosarcomas. Within this spectrum are included fibrotumefactive lesions, solitary fibrous tumors, and inflammatory pseudotumors (also called myofibroblastic tumors).

Fibromatosis

Presentation

Fibromatosis affects persons of a wide age range but involves the head and neck only 10% to 15% of the time. The symptoms vary according to location, but generally the lesion presents as a painless, enlarging mass.

Pathophysiology

The lesion is poorly circumscribed and infiltrative. Many people consider this a low-grade fibrosarcoma biologically.

Histology

Histologically, the lesion is poorly circumscribed and composed of spindle-shaped cells that have pale-staining nuclei associated with abundant collagen production. The lesion varies in cellularity and is sometimes associated with a chronic inflammatory infiltrate.

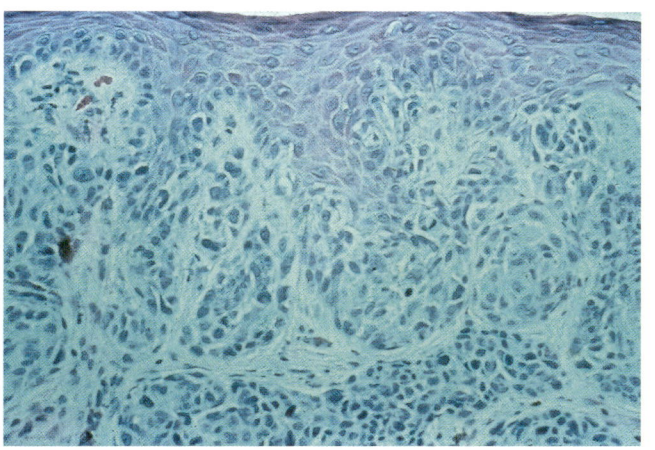

FIG. 7-5. Cutaneous melanoma.

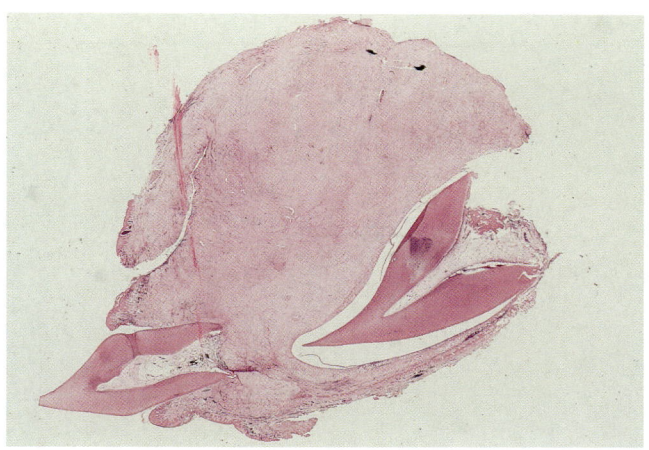

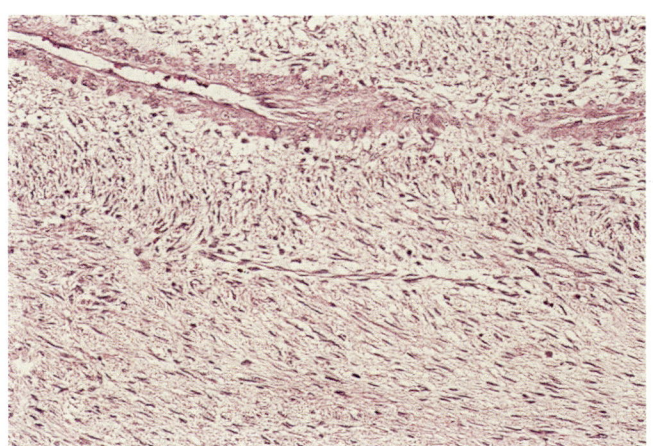

FIG. 7-7. A,B: Desmoid fibromatosis. **A** represents a central intraosseous desmoid of the jaw bone; **B** is a desmoid tumor of soft tissue.

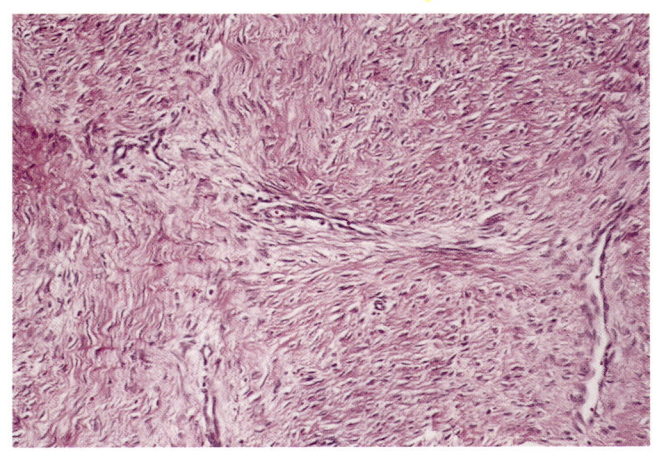

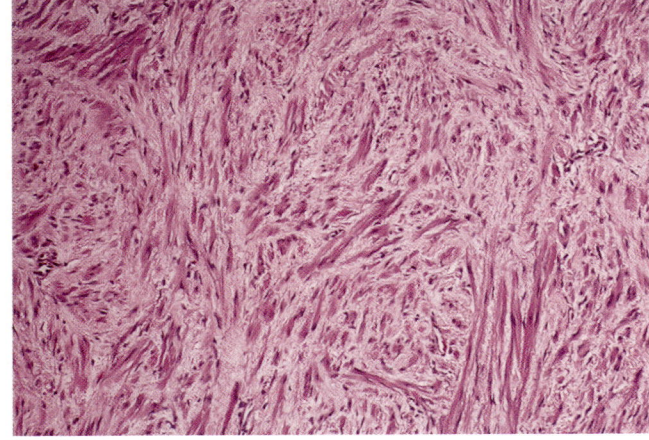

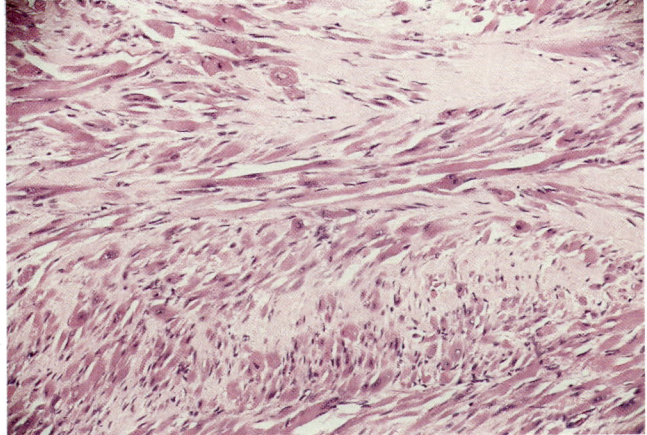

FIG. 7-6. A–C: Fibromatoses with varying degrees of cellularity.

Keloids

Presentation

A keloid usually appears as a cosmetically disfiguring scar.

Pathophysiology and Histology

Keloids result from an overabundance of dermal connective tissue, generally as a result of injury. The tendency is hereditary and most common in blacks. The exaggerated repair mechanism overgrows the area of the original injury, often to large proportions.

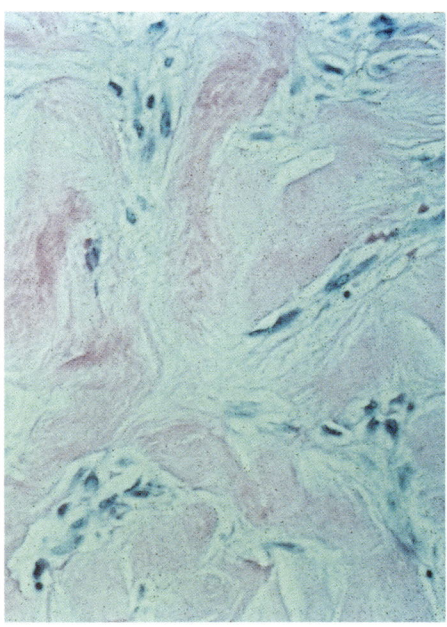

FIG. 7-8. Keloid showing markedly increased collagen deposition.

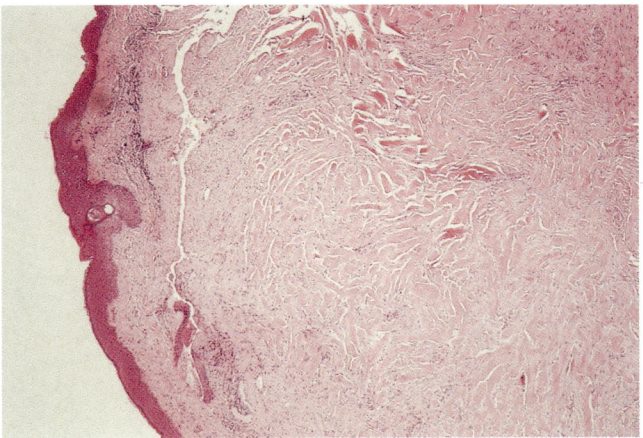

FIG. 7-9. Keloid.

Fibrosarcoma

Presentation

The sites of origin of fibrosarcomas of the head and neck in order of frequency are the soft tissues of the face and neck, the maxillary antrum, the paranasal sinuses, and the nasopharynx. Fibrosarcomas generally present as asymptomatic, slowly growing masses.

Pathophysiology

Fibrosarcomas can be divided into several types: low-grade, moderately differentiated, and poorly differentiated.

Histology

These tumors show an interwoven mixture of differentiated cells and fibers, with fibroblasts being relatively uniform in size and shape. Somewhat less differentiated tumors are more cellular and may show a "herring bone" arrangement of spindle cells. Mitoses remain sparse. Cellularity increases still further in more poorly differentiated tumors, and mitoses are frequent.

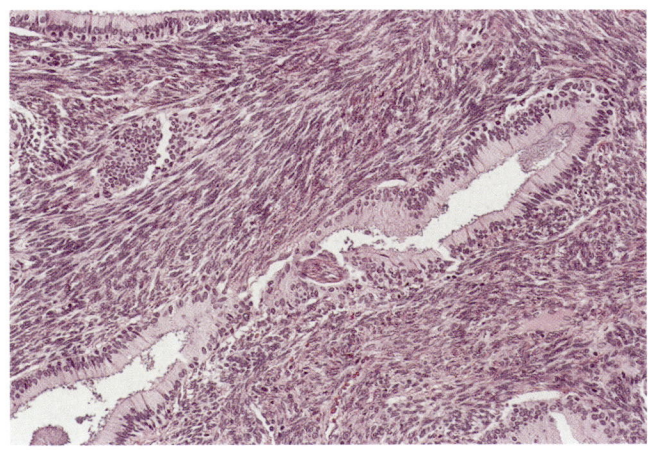

FIG. 7-10. Low-grade fibrosarcoma arising in paranasal sinus.

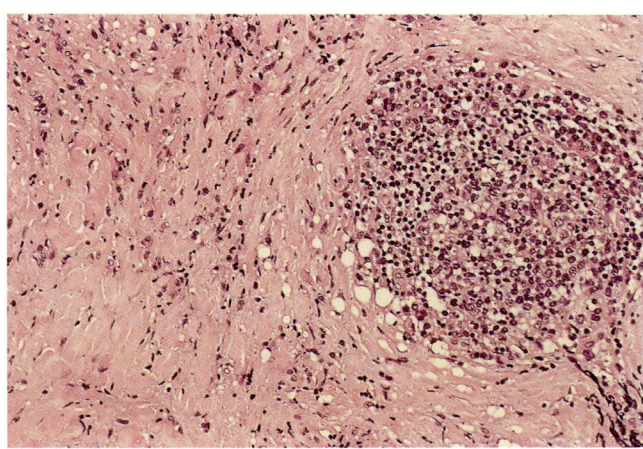

FIG. 7-11. Fibrotumefactive lesion in neck. This proliferative lesion is also known as sclerosing cervicitis, although it is not limited to soft tissues of the neck.

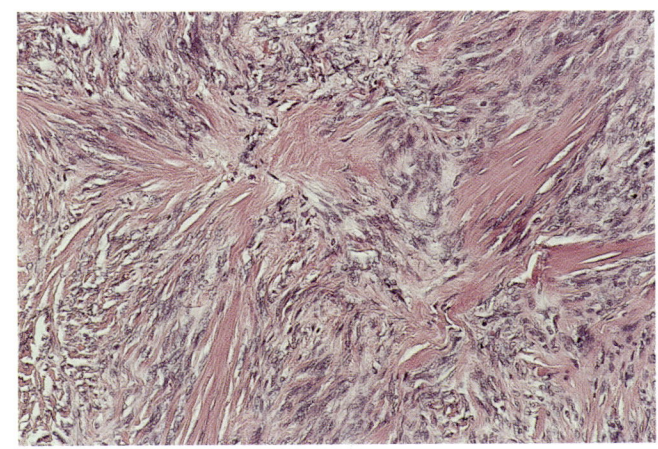

FIG. 7-12. Solitary fibrous tumor in neck soft tissues. This is the extrapulmonary version of solitary fibrous tumor of the pleura.

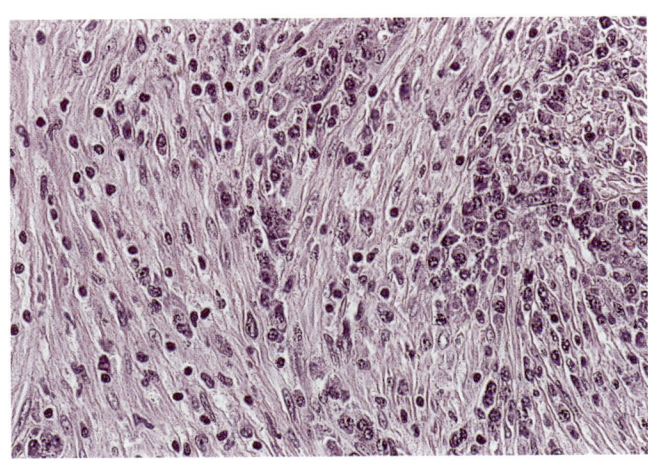
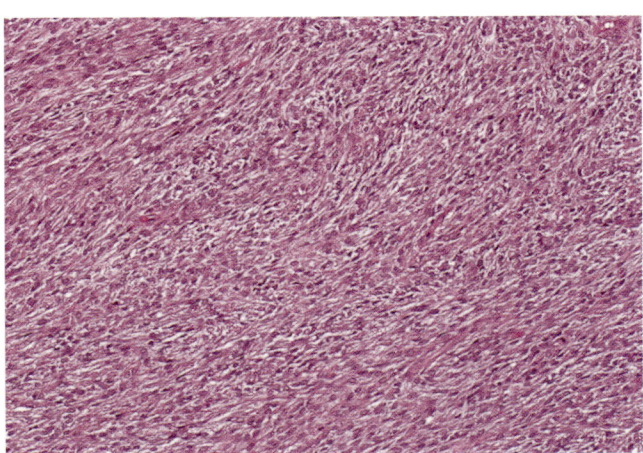

FIG. 7-13. A,B: So-called "inflammatory pseudotumor" (also called myofibroblastic tumor). In **A**, myofibroblasts proliferate with scattered chronic inflammatory cells.

Dermatofibrosarcoma
Presentation

The majority of dermatofibrosarcomas present as a nodular or multinodular mass on the scalp or neck.

Pathophysiology

Pain is variable, and for the most part these tumors are slow-growing, painless, asymptomatic masses.

Histology

The tumors usually consist of a proliferation of fibroblast-like cells, often surrounding a central acellular zone and producing a storiform (matted) pattern. In some tumors, the cells manifest an interlacing vesicular pattern. Nuclear variation is common, with the majority assuming a spindled shape. Mitotic figures may be found but are not numerous. Giant cells are rare.

MELANOMA
Presentation

Melanomas generally arise *de novo* but may also arise from a preexisting nevus, in particular a junctional nevus. This process is often heralded by a change in color, usually to dark brown or black. A fine scaling may appear on the surface of the lesion, or itching or irritation may develop in or around the lesion.

Pathophysiology

Melanoma is believed to be closely related to prior sun exposure, particularly severe sunburn. This etiology does not apply to mucosal (oral, sinonasal) melanomas. As a group, mucosal melanomas have a dismal prognosis.

Histology

Microscopically, there is invasion of the epidermis by malignant melanocytes, generally from the junctional region. Depth of invasion varies from lesion to lesion but increases over time.

HERPES
Presentation

Herpes simplex virus may infect virtually any mucous membrane but most typically infects the oral cavity. Herpes generally presents as an oral lesion that is painful.

Pathophysiology

Oral ulcers usually spontaneously subside in 5 to 7 days.

Histology

Histologically, one sees an intraepidermal vesicle with acantholysis and degeneration of the epithelial cells. Multinucleated giant cells may be seen frequently, and intranuclear inclusions may also be identified.

CANDIDIASIS
Presentation

Candida species may infect mucous membranes anywhere in the aerodigestive tract but most commonly infect the mouth, where candidiasis presents as a white, plaquelike lesion with a surrounding and underlying erythematous reaction. The lesion is usually painful.

Pathophysiology

This is usually a mucous membrane infection, often in a patient who is already ill.

Histology

Histologically, one sees the characteristic yeast with pseudohyphae.

Chapter 7/Skin and Fibrous Tissue

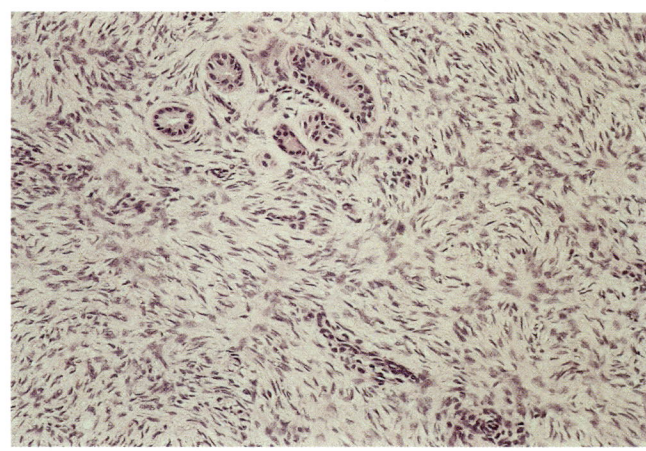

FIG. 7-14. Dermatofibrosarcoma of the skin.

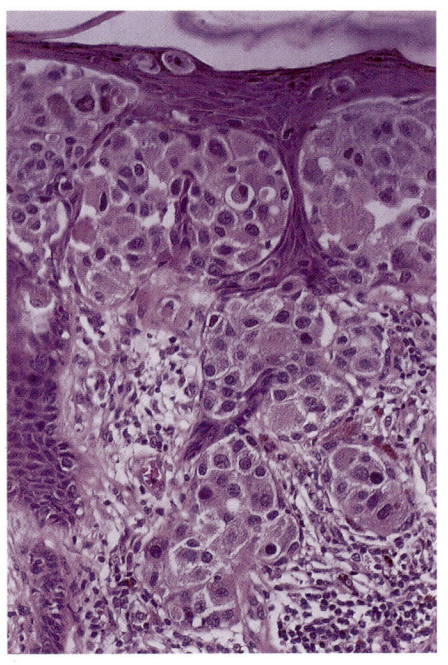

FIG. 7-15. Malignant melanoma.

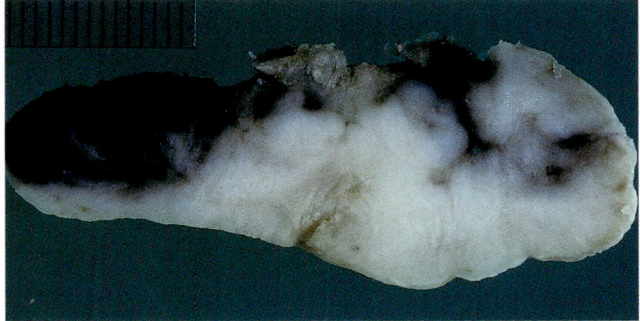

FIG. 7-16. Mucosal melanoma of the palate.

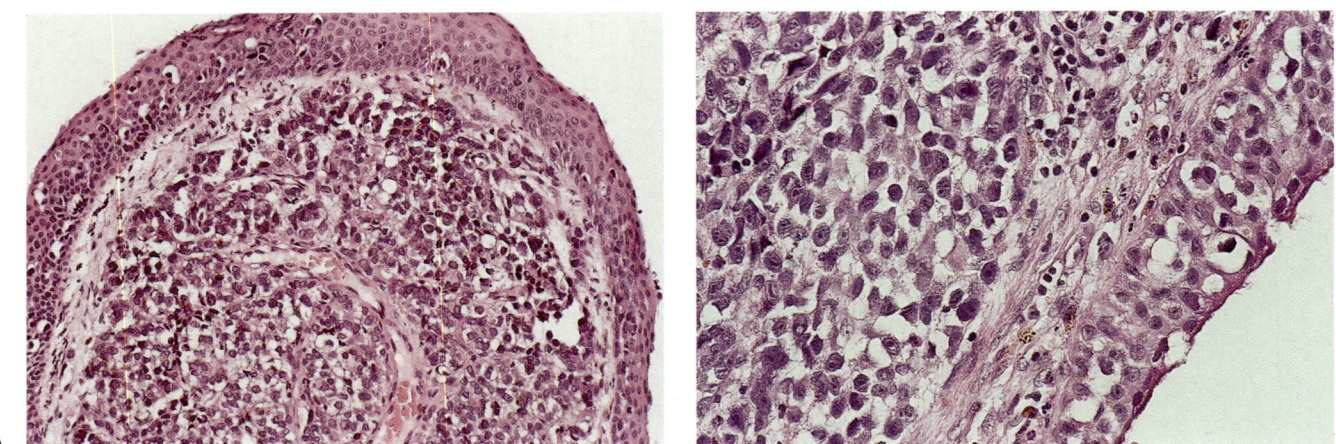

FIG. 7-17. A,B: Mucosal melanoma of the sinonasal tract.

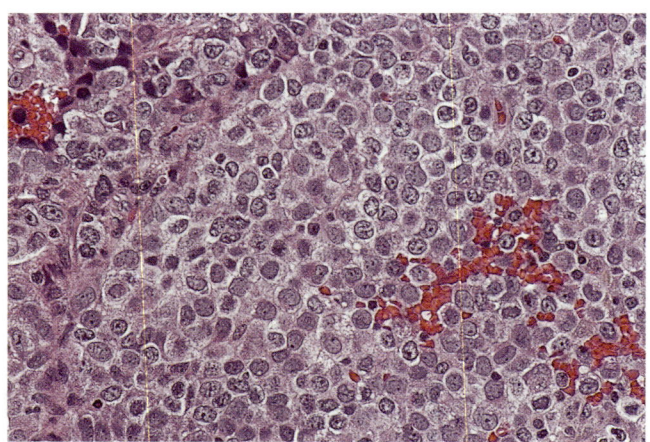

FIG. 7-18. Malignant melanoma with an epithelioid appearance.

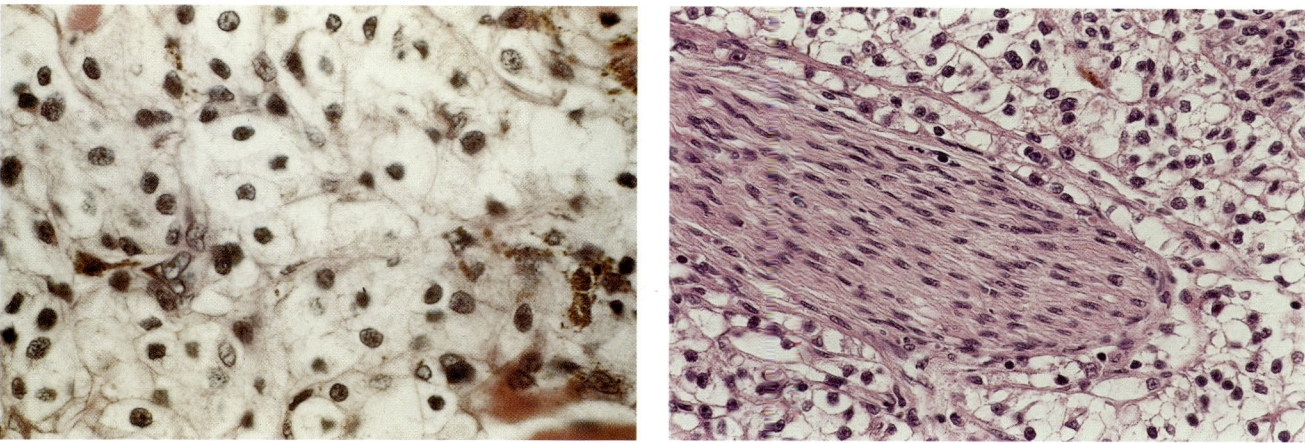

FIG. 7-19. A,B: Clear cell ("balloon") melanoma. The melanoma in **B** is from a metastasis to the parotid gland and surrounds a nerve.

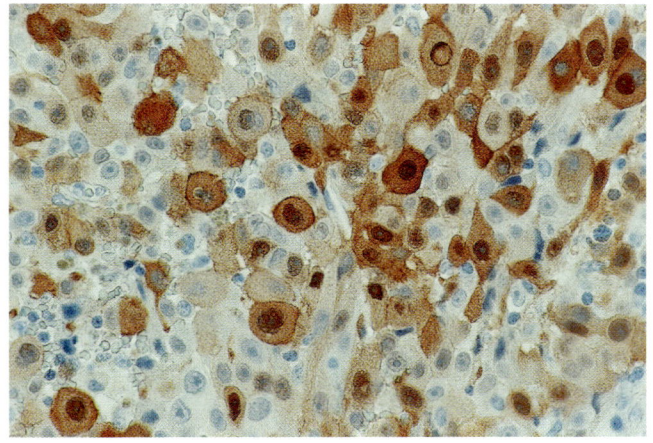

FIG. 7-20. HMB-45 immunostain of a melanoma with positive reactivity in the melanoma cells.

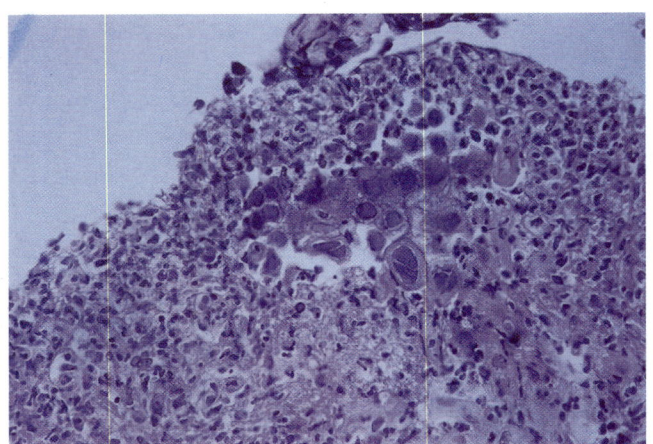

FIG. 7-21. Typical herpetic ulcer.

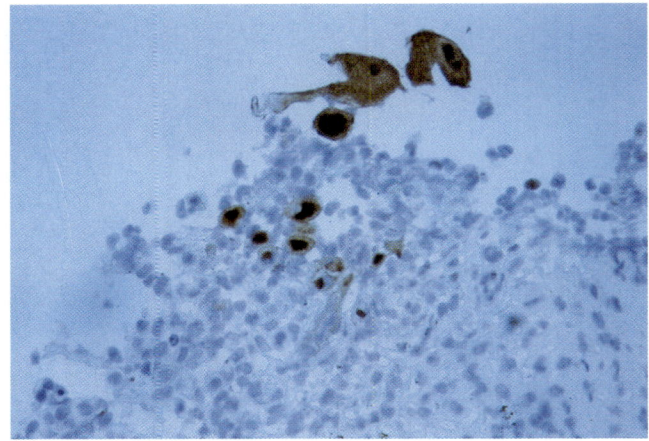

FIG. 7-22. Desquamated infected cells in herpes.

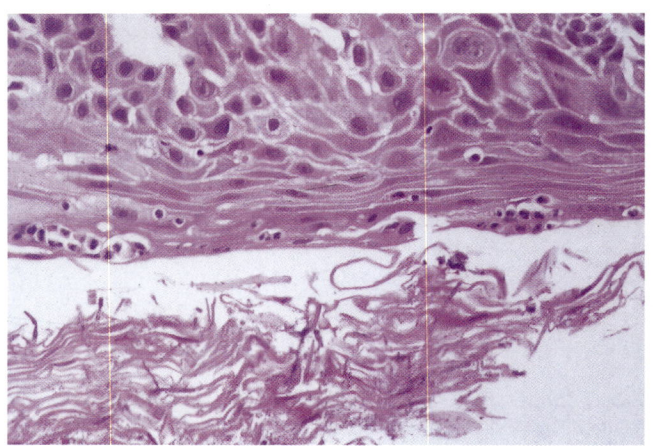

FIG. 7-23. *Candidiasis*.

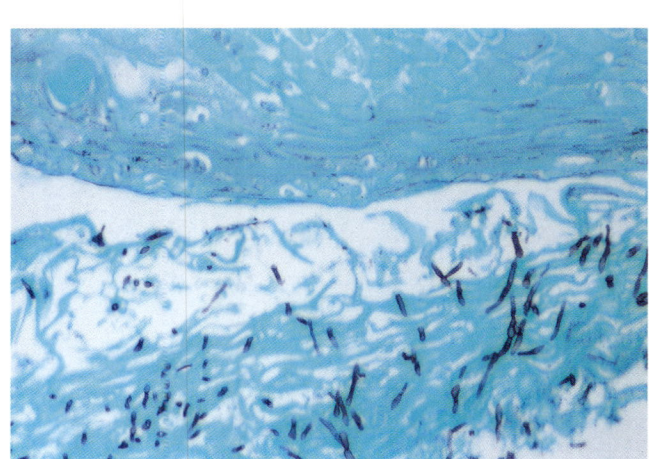

FIG. 7-24. *Candida hyphae*.

8

Dental and Bone

AMELOBLASTOMA

Presentation

The odontogenic apparatus can give rise to a bewildering array of tumors, each posing diagnostic problems, less so from a rather distinctive histologic appearance than from a limited incidence. The most common and most important is the ameloblastoma, which generally presents as a slow-growing mass.

Pathophysiology

Ameloblastomas are slow-growing, locally invasive neoplasms of the odontogenic epithelium. These tumors most commonly occur from young adulthood to middle age, with more than 80% of them situated in the mandible, usually at an angle. The tumors radiologically may be unilocular or multilocular.

Histology

This tumor in its classic form is composed of unencapsulated nests, islands, or sheets of epithelium that resemble enamel. There is a peripheral palisading of columnar or cuboidal cells with nuclei oriented away from the basement membrane. Variants may be confused with other, nonameloblastic tumors.

ODONTOGENIC KERATOCYST

Presentation

These tumors generally present as an enlarging submucosal lesion clearly involving the maxilla or, most commonly, the mandible.

Pathophysiology

Odontogenic keratocysts are felt to arise from the dental cyst that appears before the development of the dental hard tissues, and they usually are found in a location with a missing tooth. Radiologically, the cysts have well-defined radiolucent areas with a distinct margin of condensing osteitis. Multiloculation is the rule. The tumor demonstrates a locally aggressive behavior, with a 35% recurrence rate within 5 years.

Histology

The histologic features are quite characteristic. They include a thin, stratified squamous epithelium and a thin cyst wall with a paucity of inflammatory cells; "daughter" cysts may be noted in the wall. Orthokeratotic or parakeratotic layers on the surface are often accompanied by keratin within the cavity of the cysts, and variable cystic contents range from a clear to a thick, murky fluid.

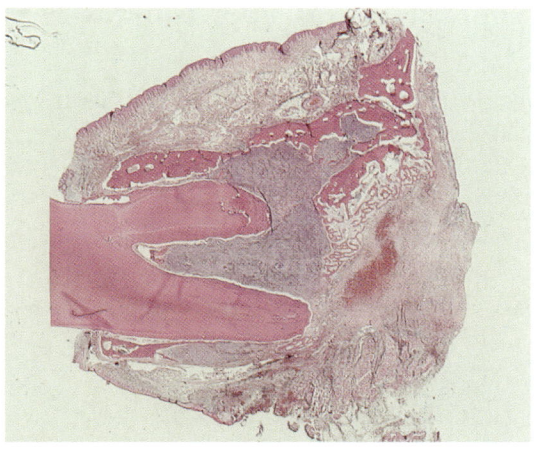

FIG. 8-1. Ameloblastoma of mandible.

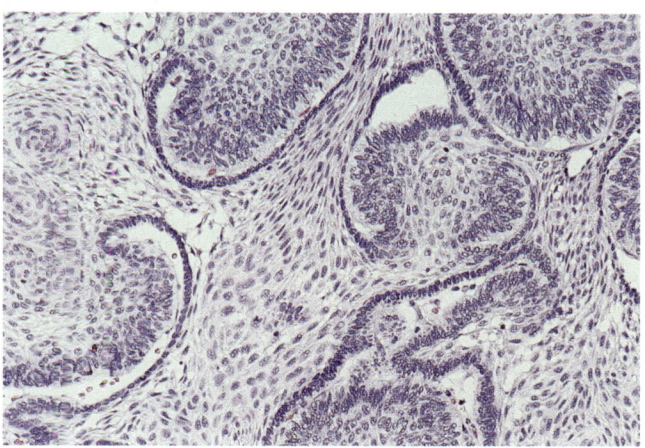

FIG. 8-2. Ameloblastoma of maxilla.

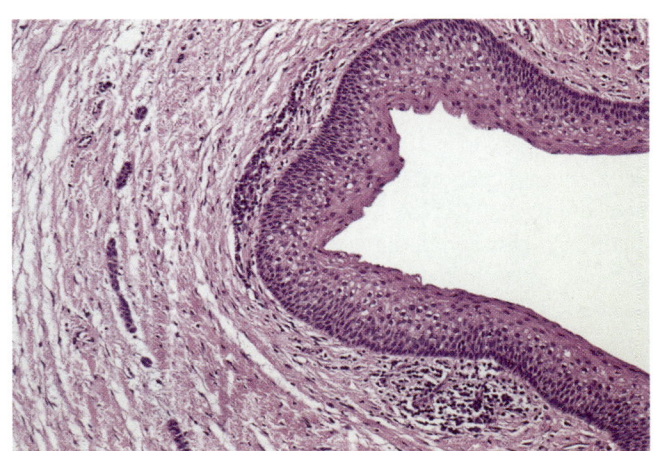

FIG. 8-3. Odontogenic keratocyst. Note near absence of a chronic inflammatory reaction.

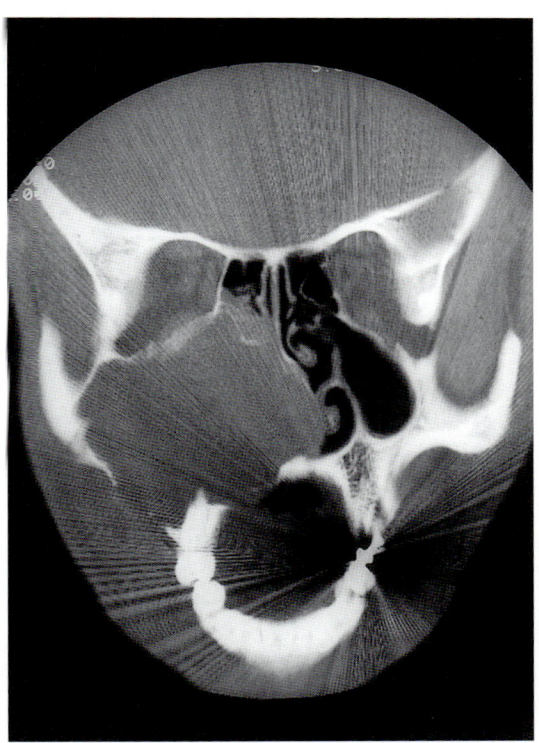

FIG. 8-4. CT scan of an odontogenic keratocyst of maxilla.

PINDBORG TUMOR (CALCIFYING EPITHELIAL ODONTOGENIC TUMOR)

Presentation

This tumor has a distinct mandibular predilection and generally presents as an enlarging submucosal mass, often in association with an unerupted tooth.

Pathophysiology

This tumor, which is quite rare, is thought to arise from enamel or dental epithelium. The tumor behaves much like an ameloblastoma, being locally invasive and locally recurrent. Radiologically, the tumor can be unilocular or multilocular, with numerous islands of irregular calcification.

Histology

There is a cellular pleomorphism with an unusual extracellular matrix and calcification. The tumor often appears as sheaths of relatively large, polyhedral epithelial cells separated by a scant connective stroma. Cytoplasm is granular and acidophilic, and intracellular bridges are found.

ADENOMATOID ODONTOGENIC TUMOR

Presentation

This tumor presents as a slow-growing submucosal mass, usually in the second decade of life, with a modest female predominance. Pain is often associated with this lesion.

Pathophysiology

This lesion is probably not a true neoplasm but more likely a developmental overgrowth of odontogenic tissue or a hamartoma. It occurs exclusively in the anterior tooth-bearing area, with 40% occurring in intimate association with an impacted tooth. Sixty percent are located in the maxilla in the incisor-cuspid area. The radiologic appearance is that of a well-demarcated unilocular radiolucency frequently associated with an unerupted or impacted tooth.

Histology

Microscopically, the tumor is well encapsulated with a central proliferation of epithelium. The cells appear to be actively secreting, and a pink, sometimes fibrillar and sometimes amorphous material is found within and between tumor cells, as well as within the lumina of ductlike structures. The tumor cells are rich in glycogen, and the material produced appears to be an acid mucopolysaccharide. It is associated with a dystrophic calcification.

SQUAMOUS ODONTOGENIC TUMOR

Presentation

This lesion presents as a painless mass, often in association with loose teeth, or sometimes as an asymptomatic expansion of the alveolar bone adjacent to a tooth. Occurrence is mainly in the second decade of life.

Pathophysiology

The tumor appears to originate from nests of Melassez in the periodontal ligament or from gingival mucosa. It is benign and rare.

Histology

Microscopically, the tumor is composed of benign squamous islands in a dense, collagenous connective tissue stroma. The epithelial islands are purely squamous in appearance. Prekeratin and keratin can be found surrounding the calcified islands.

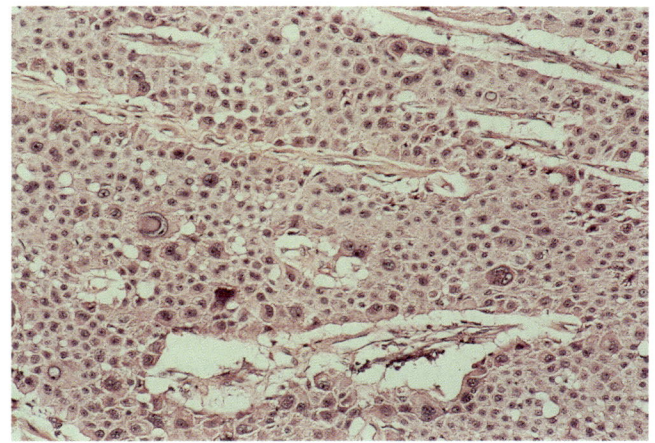

FIG. 8-5. Pindborg tumor of mandible.

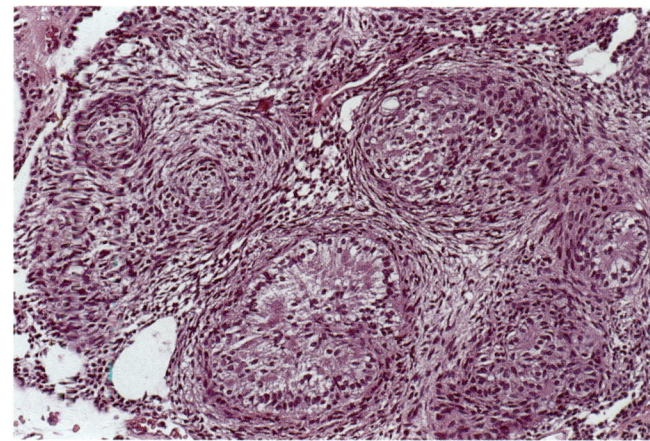

FIG. 8-6. Adenomatoid odontogenic tumor of mandible.

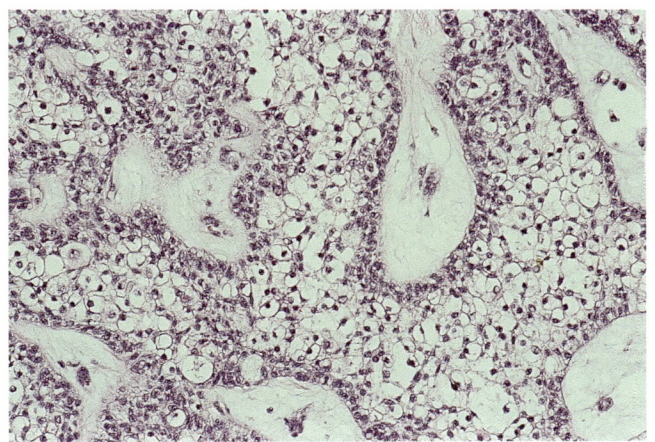

FIG. 8-7. Odontogenic clear cell tumor of mandible.

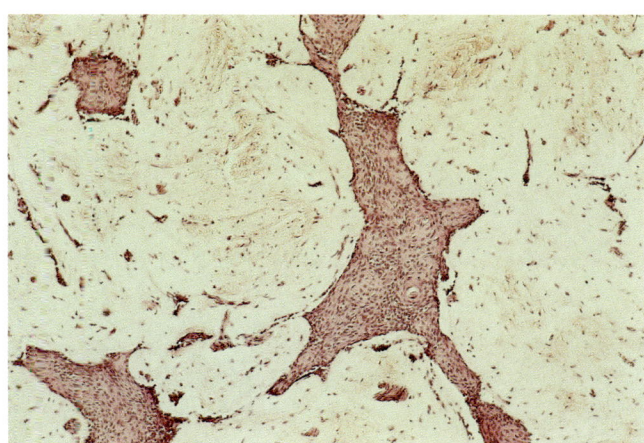

FIG. 8-8. Squamous odontogenic tumor of mandible.

ODONTOGENIC FIBROMA

Presentation

Odontogenic fibroma presents as an expanding mass.

Pathophysiology

The histogenesis of this tumor is not completely understood.

Histology

The epithelial islands in this tumor are smaller than those found in ameloblastic fibroma or ameloblastoma. Different types of calcification, including dentin, cementim, and bone, are found in varying amounts. There is a fibrous connective tissue stroma.

ODONTOGENIC MYXOMA

Presentation

This lesion occurs virtually exclusively in the mandible and presents as an expanding mass. It usually involves the posterior mandible.

Pathophysiology

The histogenesis of this tumor is poorly understood. It may arise from either dental tissues or nondental mesenchyme. Radiographically, an odontogenic myxoma cannot be differentiated from numerous other odontogenic cysts and tumors when it is small, although when larger it is multiloculated.

Histology

Microscopic examination reveals loosely arranged stellate cells within a substance rich in hyaluronic acid. This should not be confused with retained dental pulp, which will also show a circumscribed fibromyxoid connective tissue underlying degenerated odentoblasts.

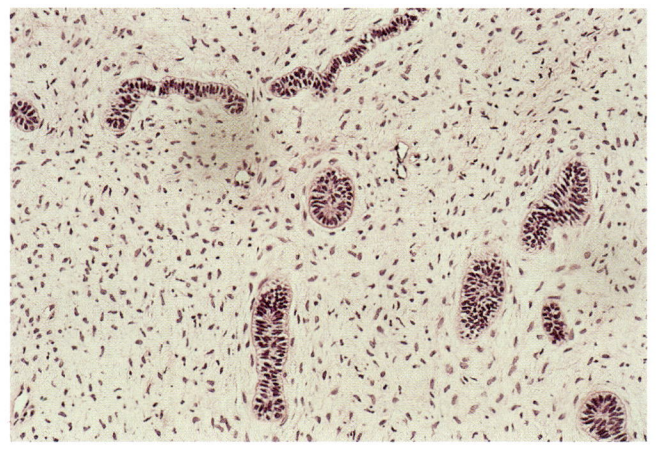

FIG. 8-9. Odontogenic fibroma of maxilla.

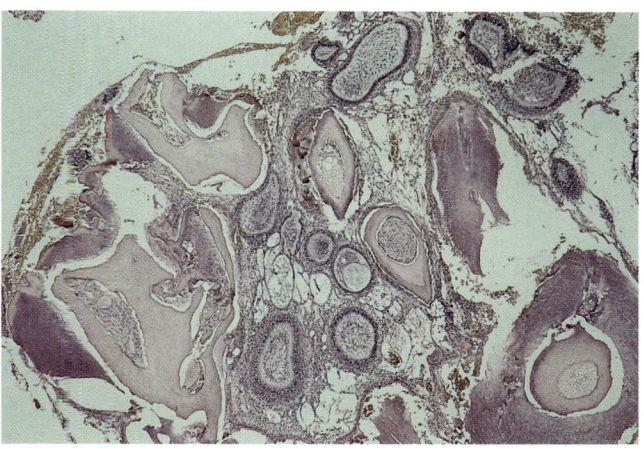

FIG. 8-10. Odontoma of mandible.

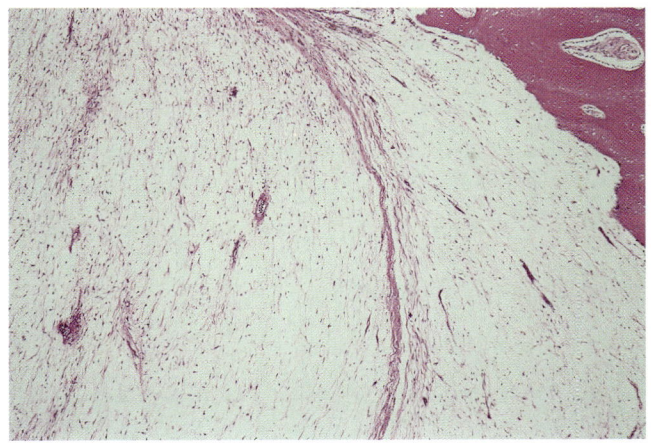

FIG. 8-11. Odontogenic myxoma of mandible.

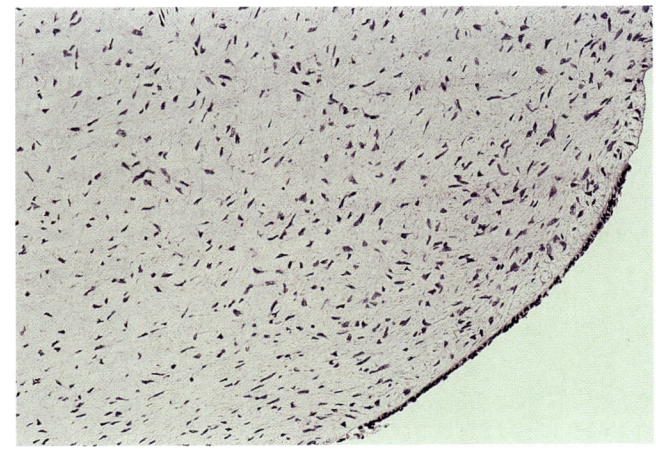
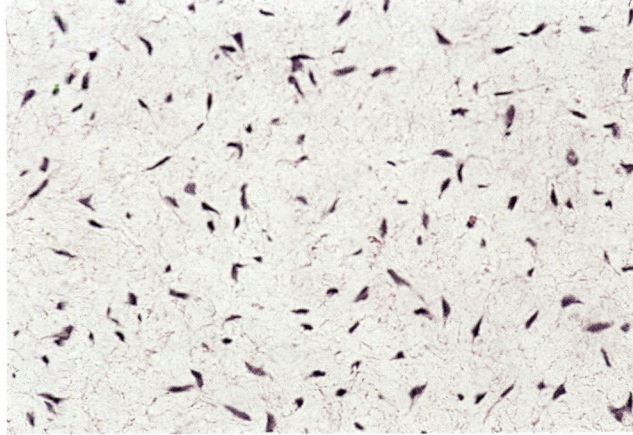

FIG. 8-12. A,B: Dental pulp. This should not be confused with odontogenic tumors such as myxoma or fibroma.

FIBROUS DYSPLASIA

Presentation

Fibrous dysplasia is twice as common in female patients and generally becomes evident in late childhood, particularly when it involves the maxilla. The presentation is one of slow, progressive facial asymmetry.

Pathophysiology

Fibrous dysplasia is a fibroosseous lesion of cryptogenic etiology in which an area of normal bone is replaced by fibrous tissue. There are three types of fibrous dysplasia: (1) involvement of a single bone (monostotic), (2) involvement of several bones (polyostotic), and (3) Albright's syndrome. The monostotic form is the most common. It typically involves the maxilla or the mandible. In the polyostotic form, the bones of the lower extremities are more commonly involved. Albright's syndrome is characterized by *café-au-lait* pigmentation of the skin, precocious puberty in female patients, and other extraskeletal abnormalities. It has a typical appearance on computed tomography, and the diagnosis can generally be made by that appearance alone coupled with the history and physical examination findings. The disease tends to be self-limiting, with progression often arrested at puberty.

Histology

Histologically, the tumor consists of an osseous component of immature bone, often misshapen trabeculae in *C*- or *S*-shaped configurations, mixed with a nondescript fibrous stroma.

OSTEOID OSTEOMA AND OSTEOBLASTOMA

Presentation

Both these lesions are benign osteoblastic neoplasms that are infrequently encountered in the head and neck. The histologic features of the two often cannot be distinguished, and the distinction is based rather on clinical aspects and size of the lesions.

Pathophysiology

Osteoid osteoma is a lesion of limited growth potential that rarely exceeds 1 cm in greatest diameter, whereas the benign osteoblastoma is larger than 1 cm and continues to grow. Sclerosis of the bone surrounding the osteoid osteoma is a distinguishing characteristic. Fewer than 20 osteoid osteomas of the jaws have been reported. Classically, osteoid osteoma is associated with pain that is worse at night and is relieved by aspirin. Similarly, osteoblastoma is quite unusual in the jaws, with also fewer than 20 cases reported, most of them in the mandible. The lesion presents with enlargement and is usually not associated with pain.

Histology

Both lesions show small, regular trabeculae of broken bone and osteoid lying in a vascular fibrous tissue. Osteoclasts are present in the fibrous tissue.

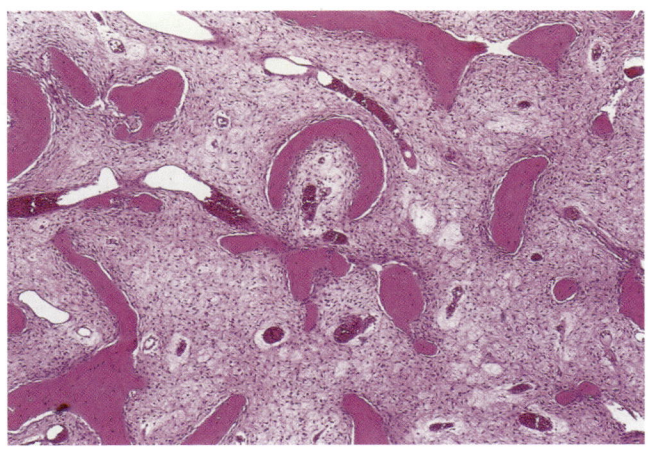

FIG. 8-13. Fibrous dysplasia of maxilla.

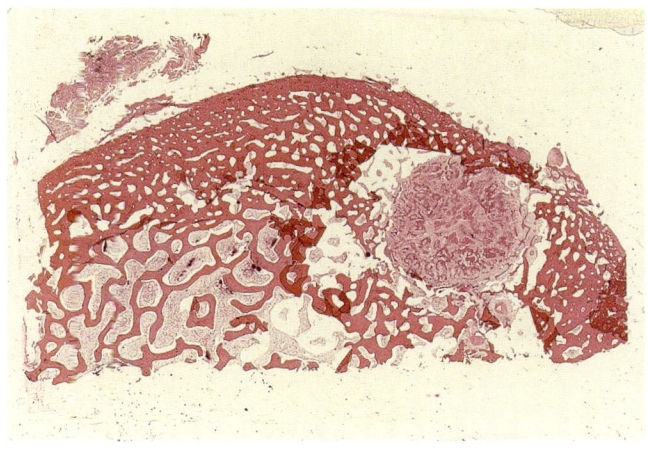

FIG. 8-14. Osteoid osteoma of mandible.

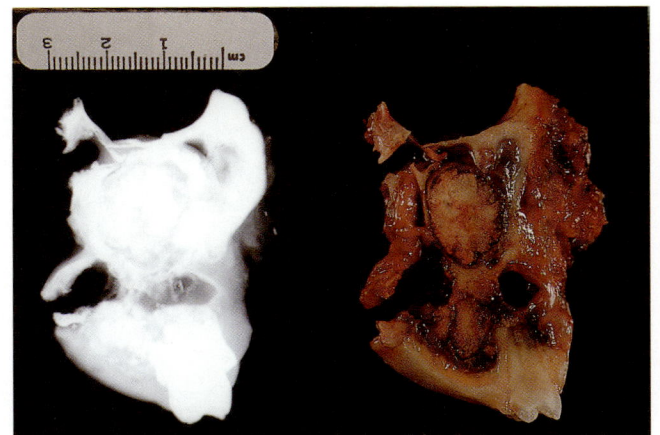
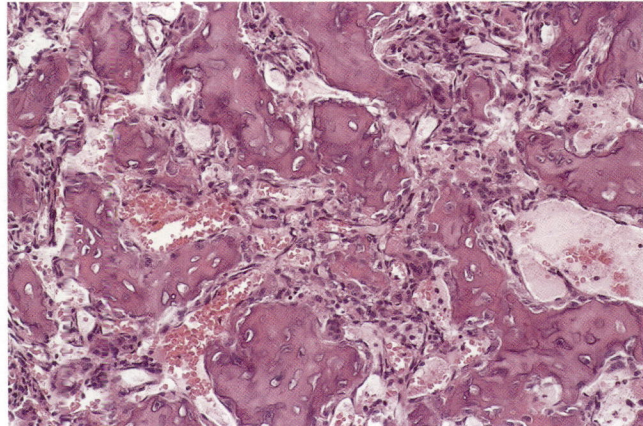

FIG. 8-15. A,B: Osteoblastoma of maxilla.

OSSIFYING FIBROMA

Presentaion

Ossifying fibroma is another benign fibroosseous lesion of bone. It most commonly occurs in the mandible as a well-circumscribed mass of fibrous tissue containing metaplastic bone. It develops most commonly in the third and fourth decades of life as a localized, nontender swelling with displacement of teeth.

Pathophysiology

Unlike fibrous dysplasia, ossifying fibroma can generally be well delineated from adjacent normal bone.

Histology

Histologically, this tumor is circumscribed and composed of mature bone spicules within a fibrous stroma. Cementifying fibroma also has a preference for the mandible and usually presents as a painless swelling of the involved bone. Cementifying fibroma may be histologically inseparable from ossifying fibroma, although there is a much greater tendency for cementem-like material to be more abundant, ovoid, and heavily calcified.

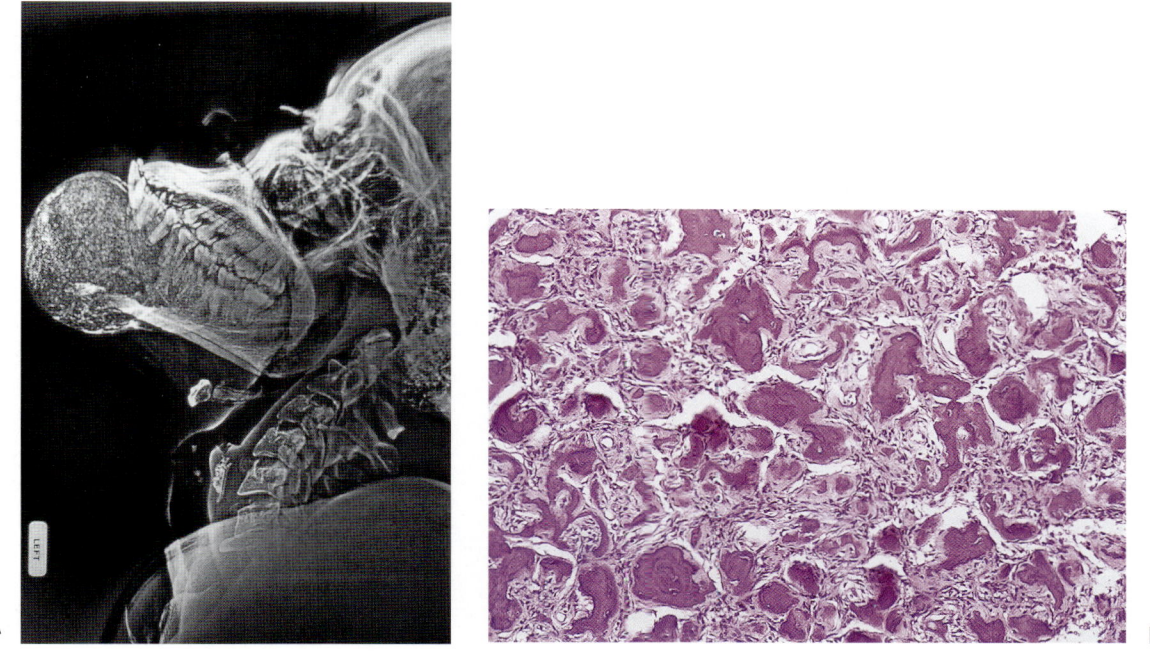

FIG. 8-16. Ossifying fibroma of mandible.

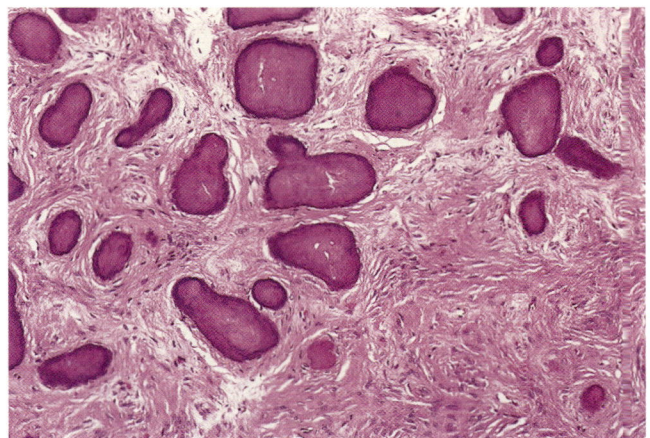

FIG. 8-17. Cementifying fibroma.

ANEURYSMAL BONE CYST

Presentation

The solitary cyst often follows a history of trauma to the area. These lesions generally present as asymmetric swellings in the bone involved.

Pathophysiology

The lesion tends to occur as an enlarging mass. It is usually not painful or tender, and the exact cause is unknown.

Histology

The histologic examination reveals meager amounts of tissue with communicating pools of venous blood in a stringy, honeycomb, fibroosseous matrix.

GIANT CELL (REPARATIVE) GRANULOMA

Presentation

Giant cell granuloma most commonly presents as an expanding lesion of the mandibular mucosa, often in an anterior position. The lesion rarely exceeds 2 cm and may be either sessile or pedunculated.

Pathophysiology

A history of trauma is often elicited, but it is not clear whether trauma is truly the etiology. The is also a peripheral (nonosseous) variant.

Histology

The histopathologic appearance is one of a proliferation of fibroblastic or mesenchymal connective tissue that is richly vascular and contains a variable number of multinucleated giant cells.

MYXOMA

Presentation

These tumors typically appear in patients in the second decade of life with an average age of approximately 30. There is a slight mandibular preference, with the tumor most commonly seen in the ramus and then in the angle of the mandible. Anterior lesions are rare. The lesions generally present as a slow-growing, asymptomatic swelling.

Pathophysiology

The origin of this tumor is uncertain and may be either odontogenic, osteogenic, both, or neither. The radiographic appearance is that of a multilocular cyst with a dense margin.

Histology

Microscopically, the tumor is characterized by polyhedral or stellate cells embedded in a soft, mucinous matrix. Nuclei are oval and often hyperchromatic. The loose, weakly basophilic stroma resembles primitive mesenchyme, with stellate cells.

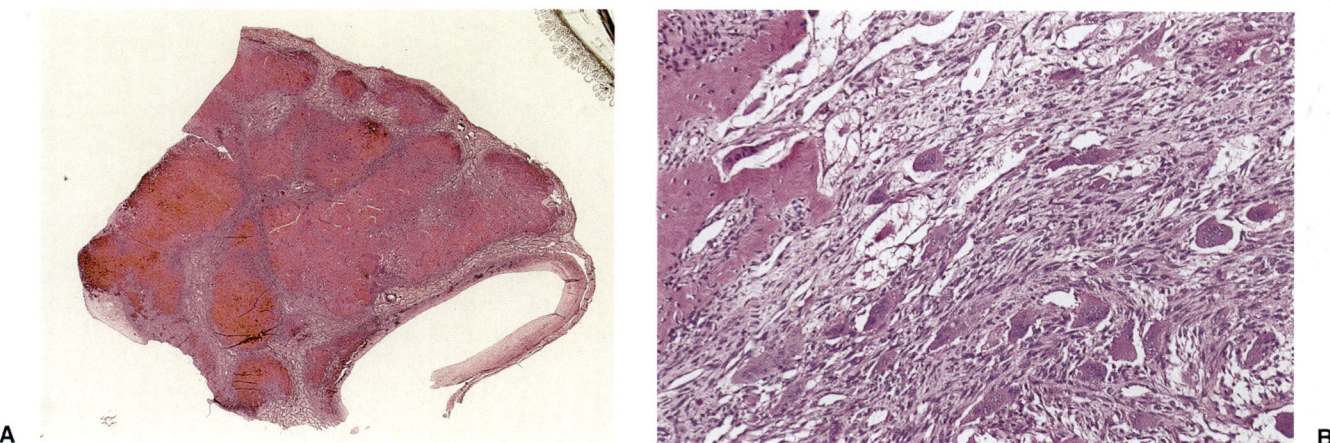

FIG. 8-18. Aneurysmal bone cyst of gnathic bone.

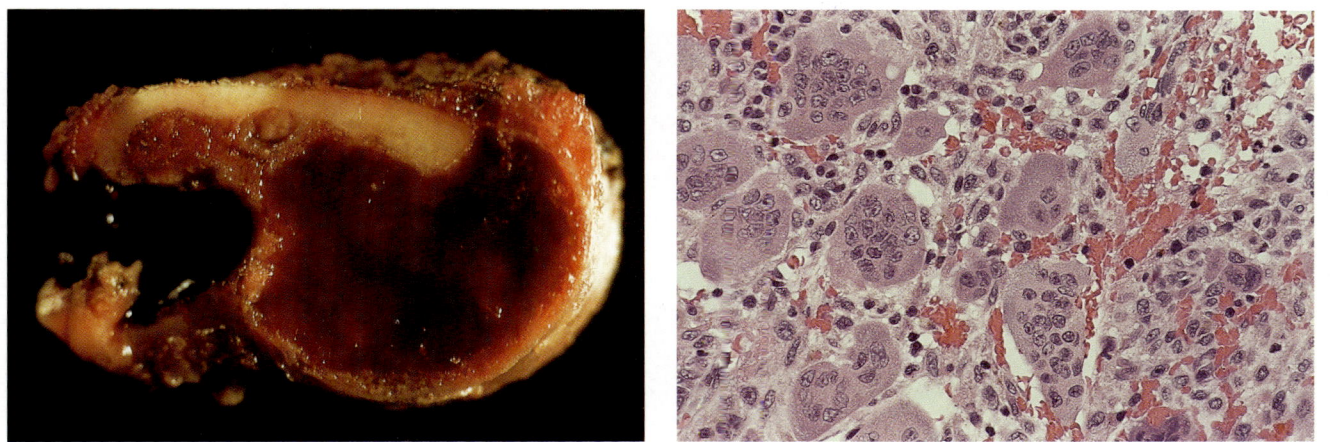

FIG. 8-19. A,B: Mandible with giant cell "reparative" granuloma.

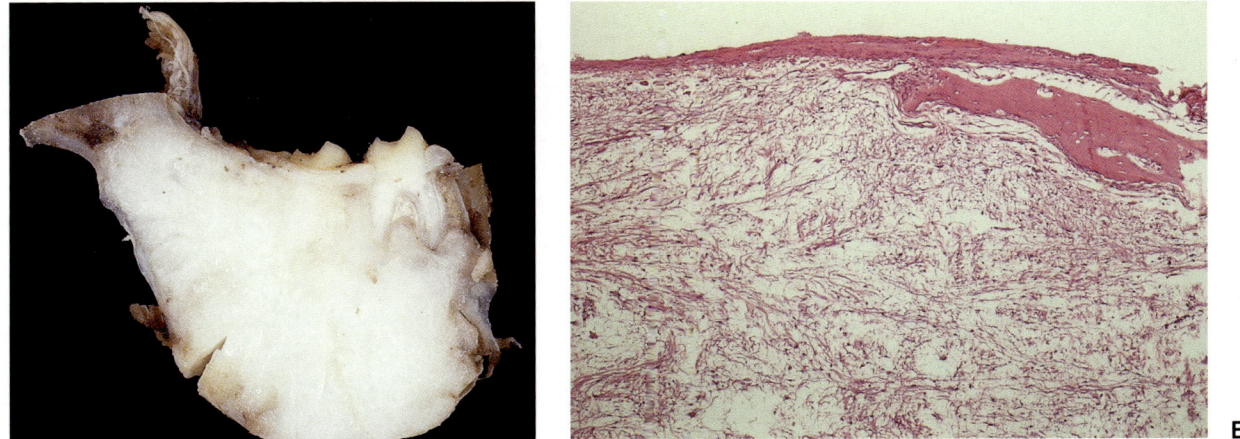

FIG. 8-20. A,B: Myxoma of mandible.

OSTEOMA

Presentation

The general presentation is that of an expanding mass that is otherwise asymptomatic. Multiple osteomas of the maxillofacial and cranial bones are a feature of Gardner's syndrome.

Pathophysiology

Osteomas are uncommon, slow-growing, benign tumors of either cancellous or cortical bone. They tend to occur in the area of the anterior ethmoidal sinus but may develop in other areas as well. The neoplasms are generally asymptomatic.

Histology

Histologically, this tumor is composed of mature, largely lamellar bone.

OSTEOCHONDROMA

Presentation

Osteochondroma usually presents as a pedunculated mass, most commonly in the tongue, head, or neck. There is a female predominance, and the tumor generally occurs between the ages of 20 and 40 years. Fewer than 100 cases have been reported in the world literature.

Pathophysiology

The tumor is an admixture of bone and cartilage. This probably represents a choristoma rather than a true neoplasm.

Histology

Microscopically, one sees a well-circumscribed lesion consisting of a mixture of mature bone and cartilage.

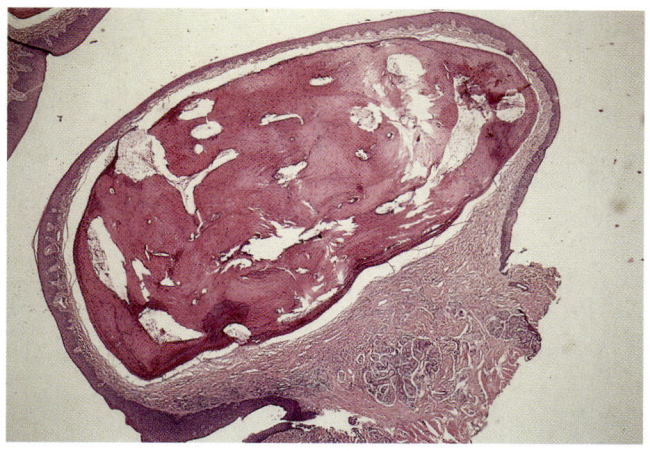

FIG. 8-21. Tongue with so-called "lingual osteoma."

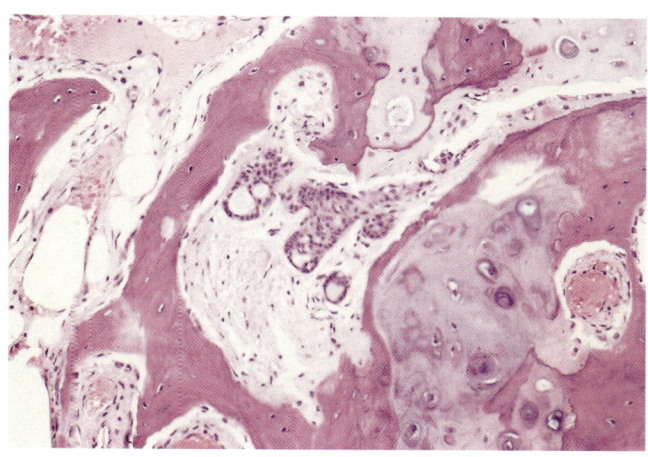

FIG. 8-22. Osteochondroma of mandible.

OSTEOSARCOMA

Presentation

Osteosarcoma is the most common malignant tumor of bone. Osteosarcomas of the head and neck occur most frequently in the second and third decades of life. These tumors generally present as localized, painless expanding masses.

Pathophysiology

The tumor is found more often in the maxilla than in the mandible. Complete excision is difficult and local recurrence common.

Histology

Histologically, one sees a sarcomatous stroma giving rise to osteoid; the stromal cells themselves display varying degrees of anaplasia, with variable pleomorphism as well.

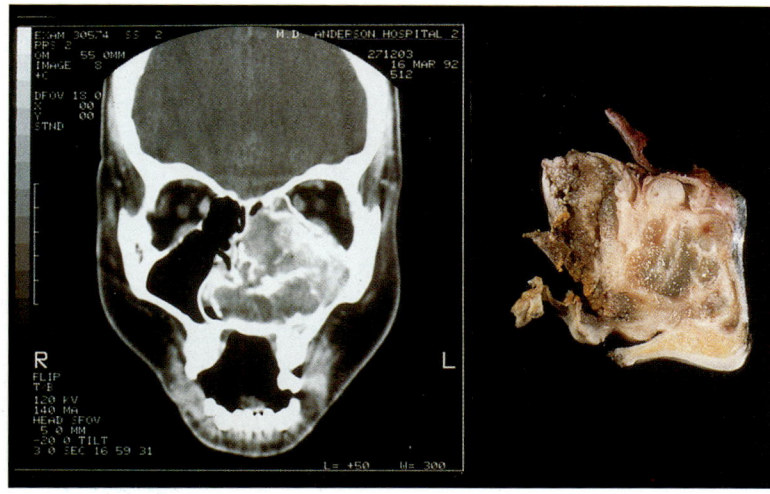

FIG. 8-23. Osteosarcoma of maxilla.

A B C D

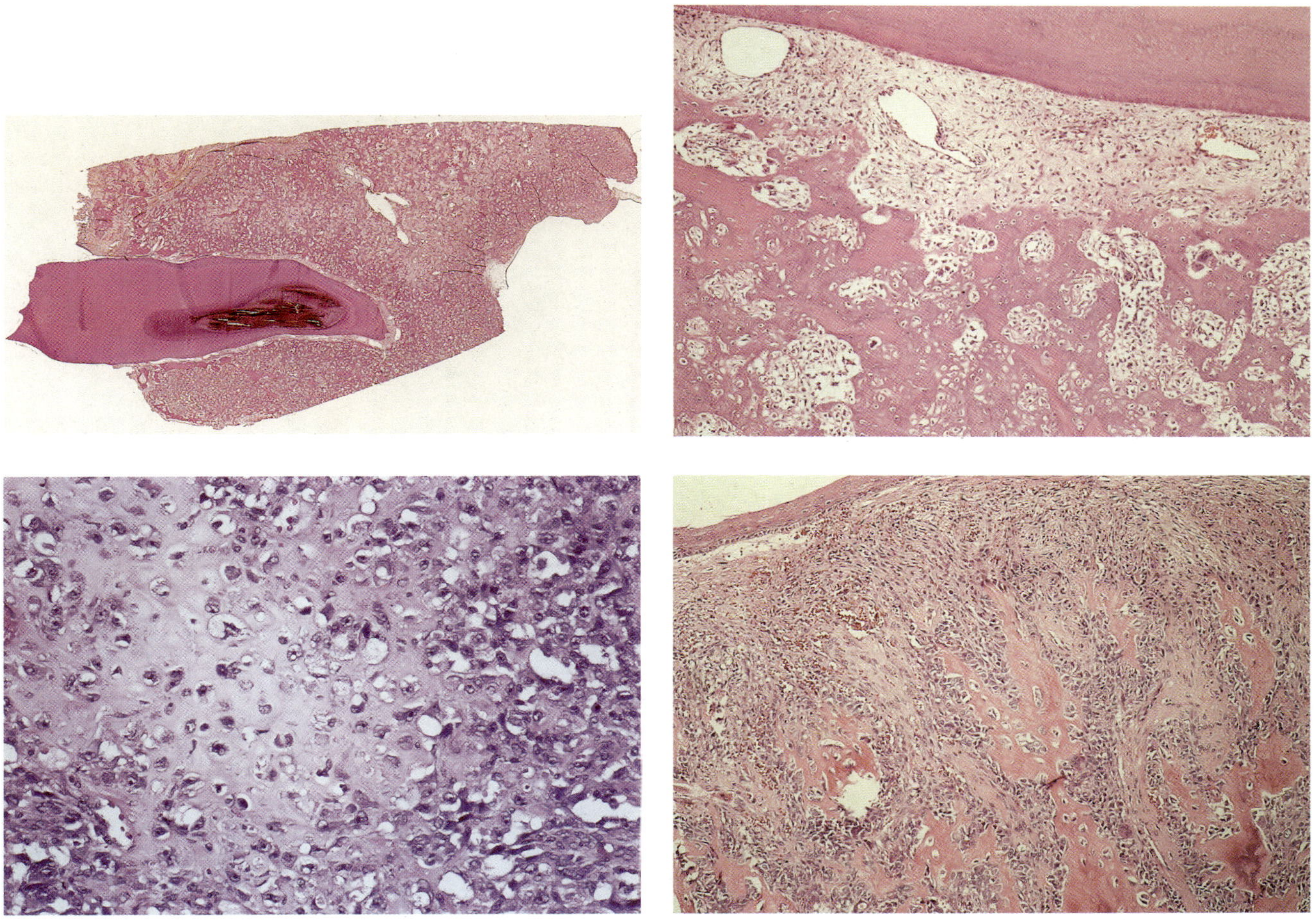

FIG. 8-24. A–D: Osteosarcomas of gnathic bones manifesting varying degrees of differentiation.

CHONDROMA AND OTHER CARTILAGE TUMORS

Presentation

Chondromas are slow-growing benign tumors of cartilage that generally manifest as a smooth, round, mucosa-covered mass.

Pathophysiology

True chondromas of the head and neck are rare and should be viewed with suspicion, particularly as most chondrosarcomas are histologically and biologically of a low grade, characterized by locally invasive behavior but limited metastatic capability.

Histology

Histologically, the tumor is composed of normal-appearing chondrocytes without pleomorphism or mitotic activity.

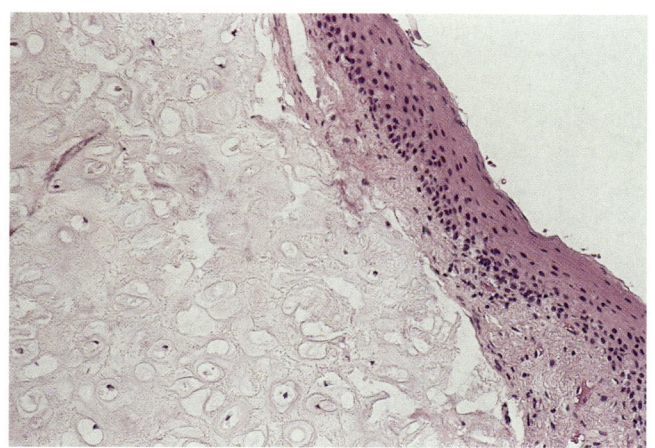

FIG. 8-25. Chondroma of epiglottis.

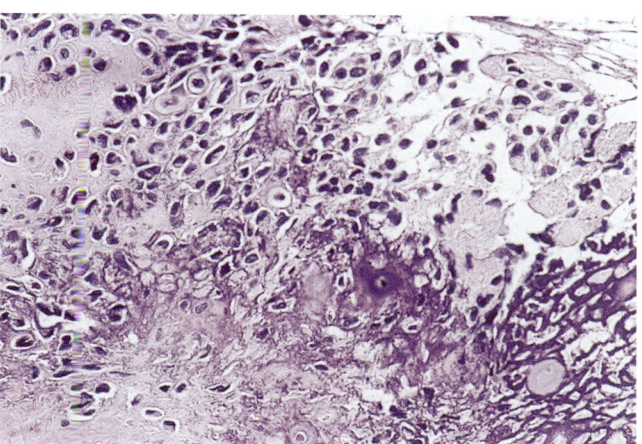

FIG. 8-26. Chondroblastoma of temporal bone.

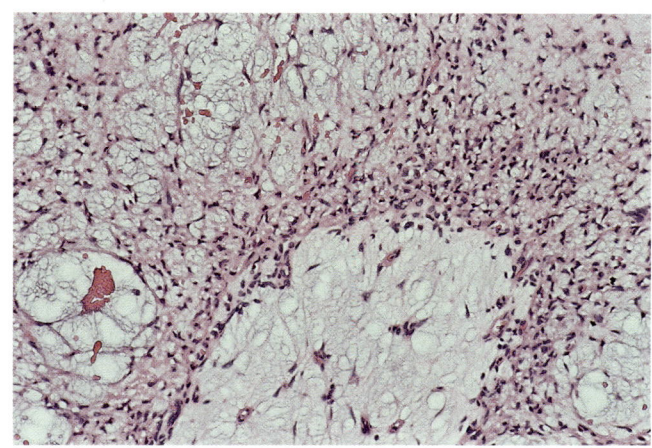

FIG. 8-27. Chondromyxoid fibroma of skull base.

CHONDROSARCOMA

Presentation

Chondrosarcoma is a malignant neoplasm of cartilage. In the head and neck, it is less common than osteosarcoma. It occurs in the mandible more frequently than in the maxilla. Unlike chondrosarcomas of the long bones, chondrosarcomas of the head and neck tend to affect patients in their fifth or sixth decades. The tumors generally present as painless expanding masses. In the larynx, chondrosarcomas can be mistaken for chondromas because of their low-grade histology.

Pathophysiology

The prognosis is poor because of relentless local recurrence.

Histology

Histologically, the tumor is hypercellular. Hyperchromatic and pleomorphic nuclei are apparent, and multinucleated cells may be present. Generally, these tumors are given a low or high grade depending on the degree of cellularity, but the majority are of a low grade.

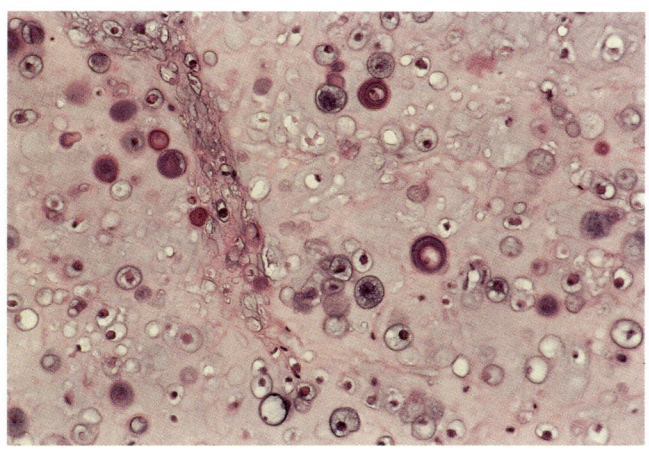

FIG. 8-28. Chondrosarcoma of maxilla.

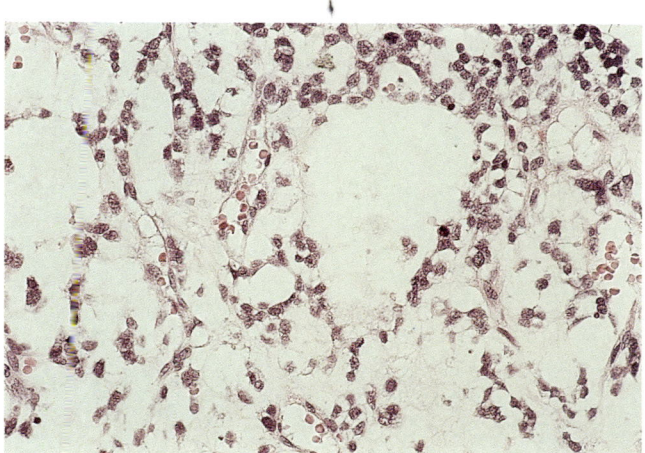

FIG. 8-29. Myxoid chondrosarcoma of skull base.

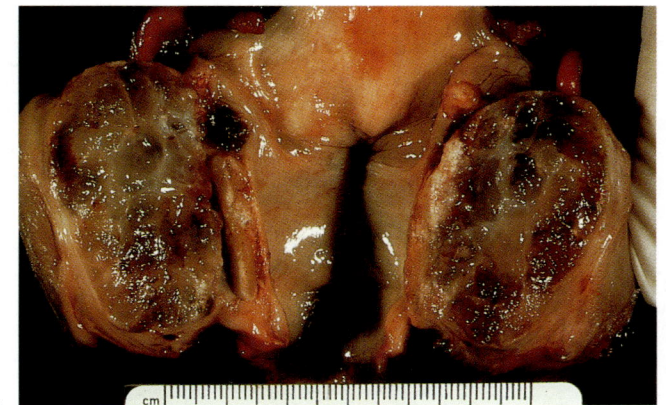
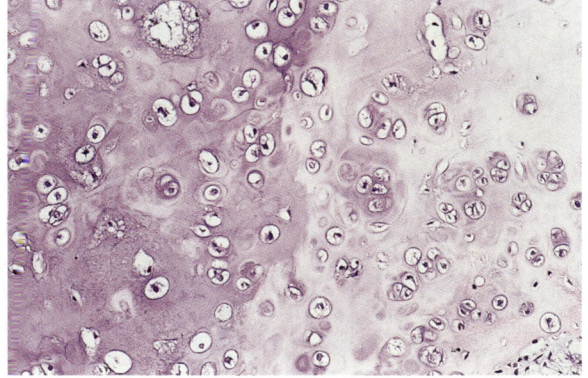

FIG. 8-30. A,B: Chondrosarcoma of larynx.

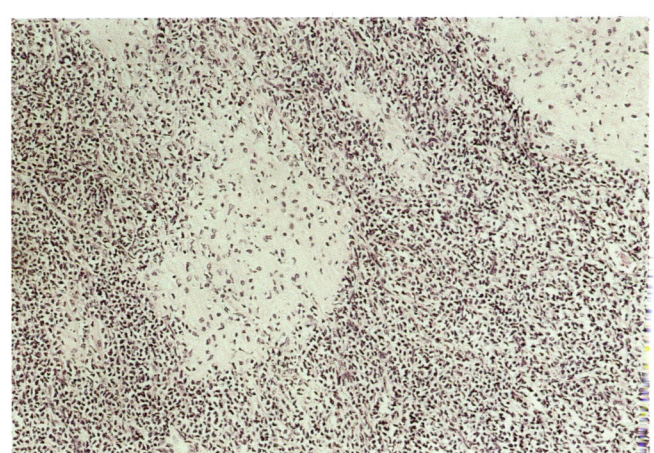

FIG. 8-31. Mesenchymal chondrosarcoma of maxilla.

CHORDOMA

Presentation

Chordomas in the head and neck generally occur at the base of the skull, with the majority arising in the region of the clivus. Chordomas may occur at any age, but the peak incidence is between the ages of 20 and 40. Patients usually present with neuroophthalmologic and otologic symptoms resulting from involvement of the cranial nerves. Headache is a nearly constant feature.

Pathophysiology

This tumor is dysontogenetic and appears to arise from vestigial remnants of the embryonic notochord.

Histology

There are no absolute or specific histologic features, but four findings are fairly constant: (1) overall lobular arrangement of cells; (2) tendency of cells to grow in cords or irregular bands, or in a pseudoacinar form; (3) production of an abundant intercellular mucinous matrix; and (4) presence of large physaliphorous and vacuolated cells.

PAGET'S DISEASE

Presentation

Paget's disease is a rare idiopathic affliction of the adult skeleton that generally appears between the fourth and sixth decades of life. The incidence increases with advancing age. Many cases, however, are subclinical. The disease generally presents as gradual enlargement of the jaws, resulting in a spreading of the teeth and disordered occlusion. Retroclination of the incisor teeth and palatoversion of the posterior teeth are constant and striking features.

Pathophysiology

Idiopathic deformation of affected bone leads to significant weakening of bone, although fractures in the jaws are uncommon. Because of extensive arteriovenous communications, involved areas are characteristically warmer than surrounding, unaffected areas. Radiographically, osteoporosis is an early finding, with a "cotton-wool" appearance developing later.

Histology

Microscopically, during the early phases, one sees large quantities of new bone in a loose, vascular, connective marrow. Later, simultaneous osteoblastic and osteoclastic activity is apparent.

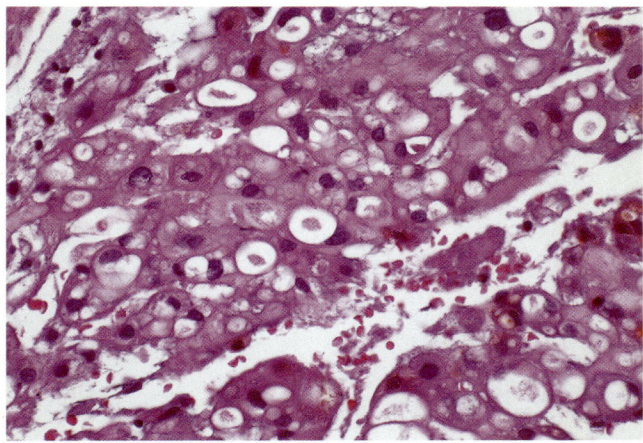

FIG. 8-32. Chordoma of skull base.

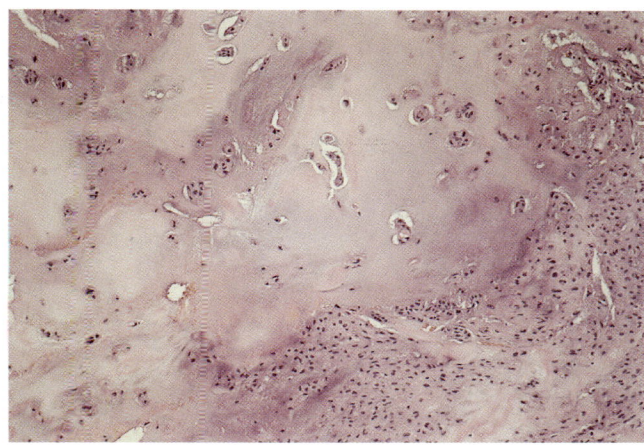

FIG. 8-33. Chordoma showing chondroid foci, so-called "chondroid chordoma."

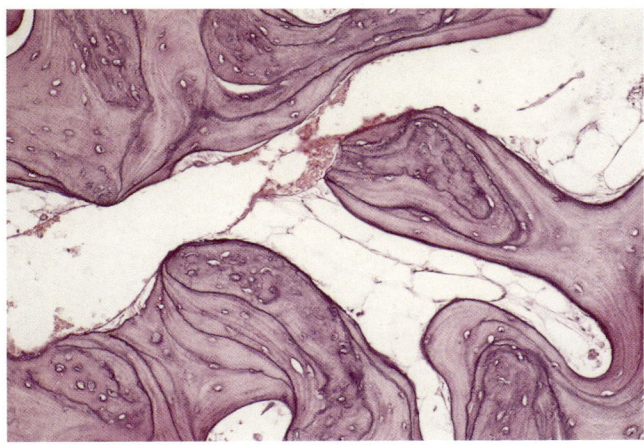

FIG. 8-34. Paget's disease of bone in mandible.

PART II

Non–site Specific Diseases

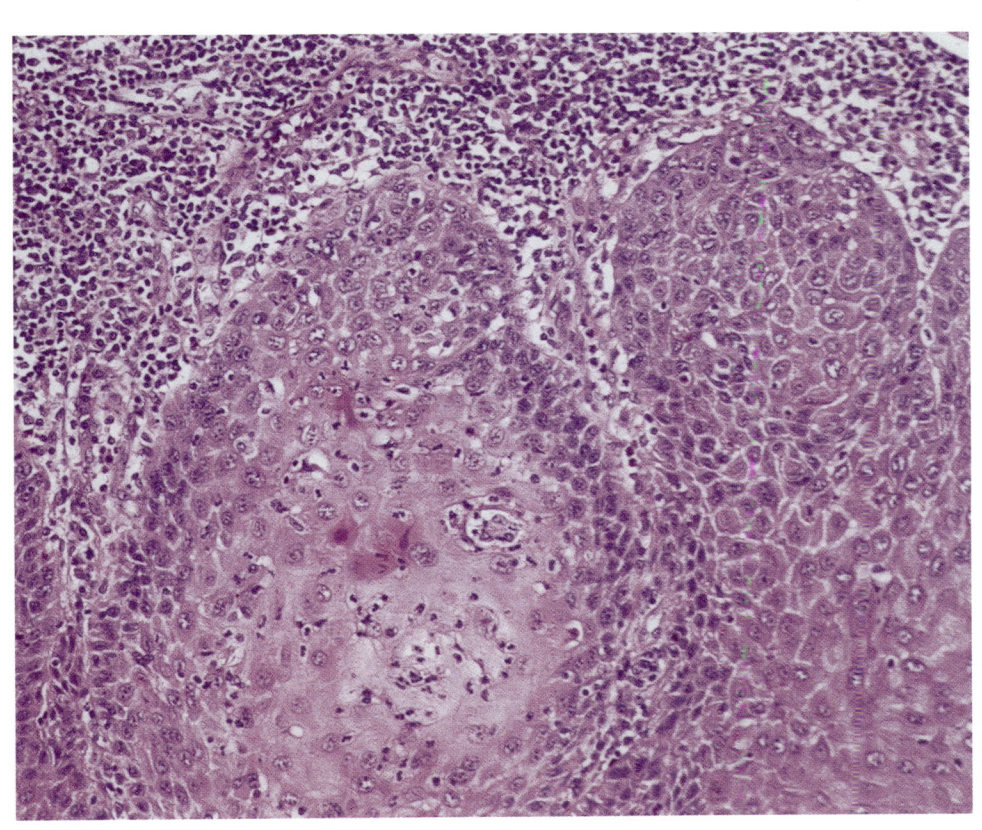

9

Inflammatory Lesions

MYCOBACTERIAL INFECTIONS

Presentation

Symptoms vary depending on the site involved, but the most common manifestation is site-specific. Infection is usually manifested by unilateral cervical adenopathy that is generally not tender.

Pathophysiology

Mycobacterial infections of the head and neck may be caused by a variety of mycobacteria, but most commonly *Mycobacterium tuberculosis* or one of the atypical mycobacteria. The infections may involve the lymph nodes, tonsils, sinus and nasal cavities, pharynx, oral cavity, larynx, salivary glands, or temporal bone.

Histology

Histopathology of the lesions will show caseating granulomas, but the bacterium itself may or may not be identified, so that culture confirmation is required.

CAT-SCRATCH DISEASE

Presentation

Cat-scratch disease is a relatively common cause of cervical adenopathy that might be mistaken for bacterial or mycobacterial adenitis. The causative agent is now thought to be a pleomorphic gram-negative bacillus that can be seen with the Warthin-Starry silver impregnation stain.

Pathophysiology

The adenopathy is often tender. There is no sex or age predilection. The mode of transmission is by direct contact.

Histology

Histologic changes vary from hyperplasia with a histiocytic proliferation to a granulomatous stage and may progress to abscess formation.

RHINOSCLEROMA (SCLEROMA)

Presentation

Rhinoscleroma is endemic to subtropical countries in Africa, Asia, South and Central America, and eastern Europe. In the United States, it is seen more frequently in the southwest and western regions and where hygiene is poor. The causative agent is *Klebsiella rhinoscleromatis*. The infection almost always starts in the nasal cavity but may extend down into the larynx and trachea. It generally begins as a firm submucosal plaque that expands into a hard nodule; depending on location, this may cause airway obstruction.

Pathophysiology

As the disease progresses, fibrosis and scarring increase.

Histology

Histologically, one sees a submucosal granulomatous infiltrate composed of macrophages that have a foamy cytoplasm (Mikulicz's cells) associated with a mixture of lymphocytes and plasma cells. The overlying epithelium may demonstrate pseudoepitheliomatous hyperplasia. Macrophages ingest the bacteria, which may be seen with the Warthin-Starry stain. Gram's stain may also reveal the organism.

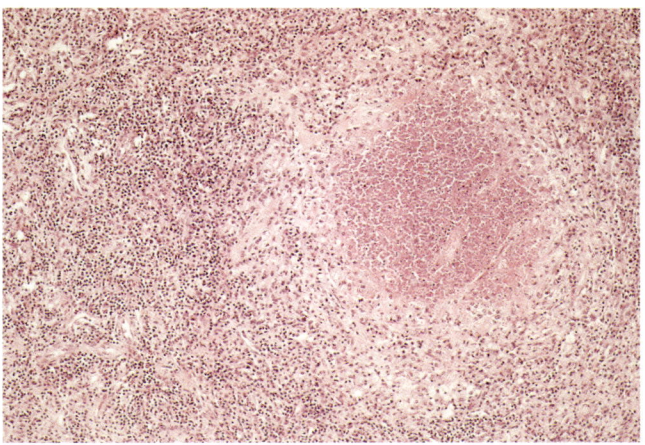

FIG. 9-1. Cat-scratch disease in a cervical lymph node.

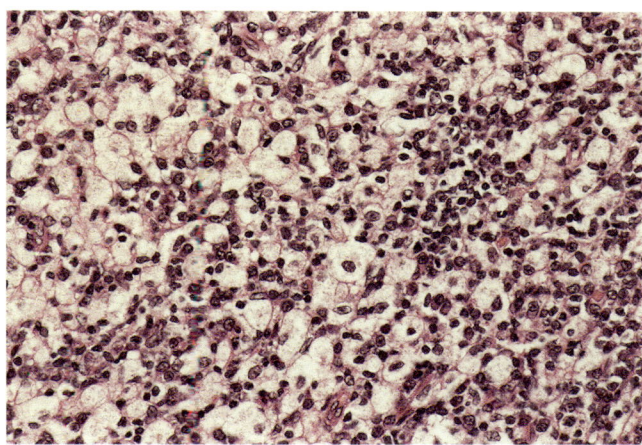

FIG. 9-2. Rhinoscleroma in the nasal mucosa. Note the vacuolated foamy macrophages (Mikulicz's cells).

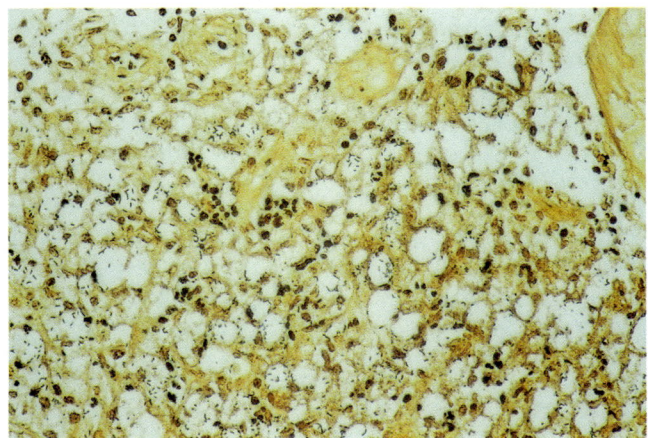

Fig. 9-3. Rhinoscleroma stained to demonstrate intracellular *Klebsiella rhinoscleromatis* organisms.

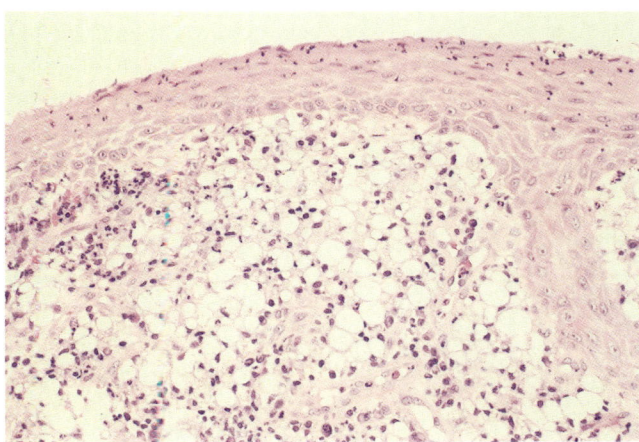

FIG. 9-4. Photomicrograph showing a submucosal granulomatous infiltrate composed of macrophages with foamy cytoplasm in rhinoscleroma.

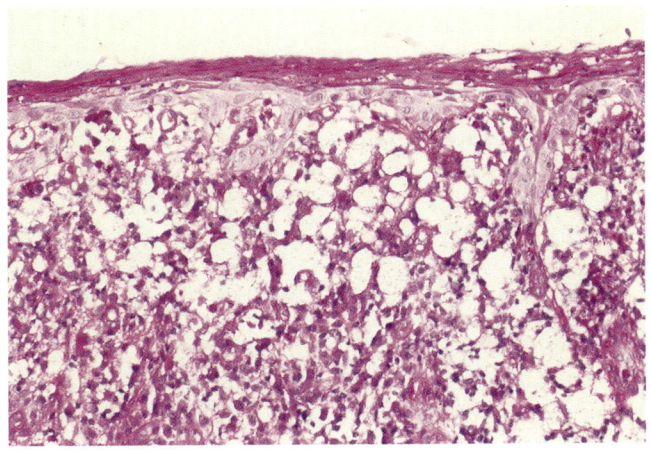

FIG. 9-5. Rhinoscleroma.

RHINOSPORIDIOSIS

Presentation

Rhinosporidiosis is a granulomatous disease caused by the fungus *Rhinosporidium seeberi*. It is endemic to poor areas in Sri Lanka, Africa, and India, and commonly presents in young male adults from India with an irregular, dull pink to red polyp or mass that bleeds and is friable.

Pathophysiology

Nasal obstruction, epistaxis, and purulence are common symptoms. Squamous metaplasia may overlie these lesions.

Histology

Histologically, one sees submucosal cysts ranging in size from 10 to 300 μm in diameter. The cysts contain endospores that may be seen by hematoxylin and eosin stain. The organisms may also be seen with period acid–Schiff and mucicarmine. The chronic inflammatory response consists of leukocytes and plasma cells with eosinophils.

LEPROSY

Presentation

Leprosy is endemic to warm, medically deprived areas. The causative agent is *Mycobacterium leprae*. This organism tends to attach to subcutaneous nerves and secondarily to the skin and mucosa of the upper respiratory tract. Occasionally, cases occur in the southern parts of the United States, with two principal forms of the disease.

Pathophysiology

Tuberculoid leprosy is a relatively benign and self-limiting form affecting people who are relatively resistant to the offending organism. On the other hand, lepromatous leprosy, a disseminated form, occurs in patients with low resistance. In this case, the bacterium may be found in all tissues of the body. The bacterium has been successfully grown only in the armadillo.

Histology

Histologically, there are noncaseating granulomas with numerous large foam cells. The foam cells (histiocytes) contain the bacteria, which can be demonstrated by acid fast stains.

BLASTOMYCOSIS

Presentation

The patient usually presents with a cough and a low-grade fever. A cutaneous verrucous lesion with a serpiginous border is generally seen.

Pathophysiology

This disease, caused by the fungus *Blastomyces dermatitidis*, is quite rare in the United States. It occurs in South America and Africa. In North America, blastomycosis is most commonly found in the Missouri, Mississippi, and Ohio River Valley areas. It typically affects the pulmonary system, although hematogenous spread may lead to wide dissemination.

Histology

The lesions are characterized by acute and chronic inflammation, microabscesses, and giant cells. The overlying epithelium may show pseudoepitheliomatous hyperplasia. Fungal stains will show the organism in its yeast form.

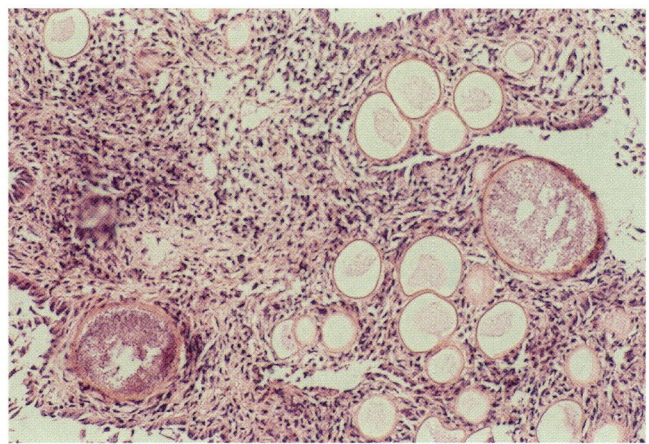

FIG. 9-6. Rhinosporidiosis in nasal cavity.

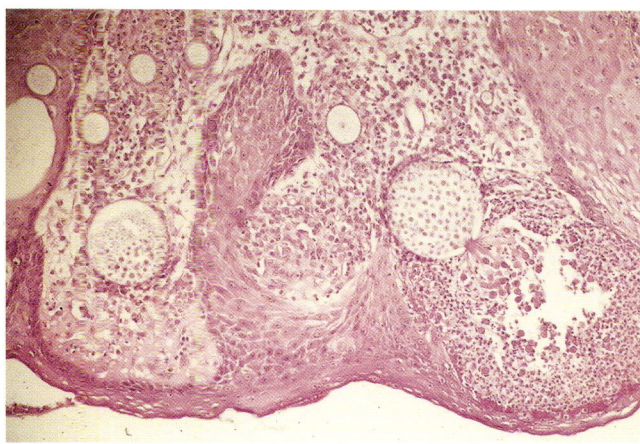

FIG. 9-7. Rhinosporidiosis showing a chronic inflammatory response with leukocytes, plasma cells, and eosinophils.

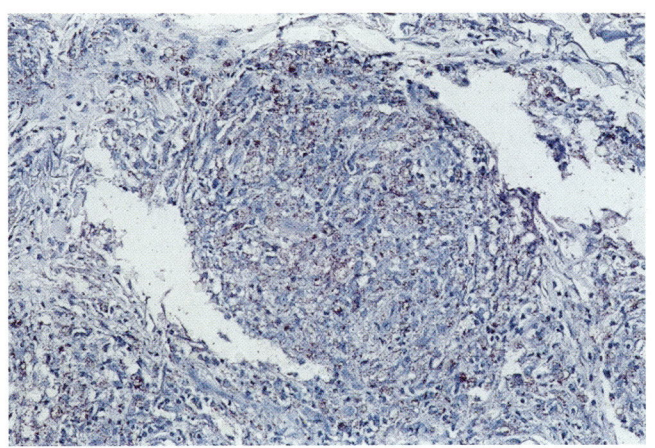

FIG. 9-8. *Mycobacterium leprae* (Hansen's bacillus) in a nasal granuloma.

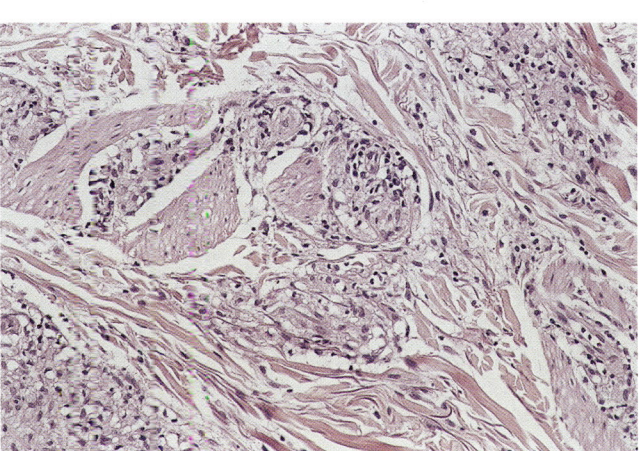

FIG. 9-9. Leprosy with perineural granuloma.

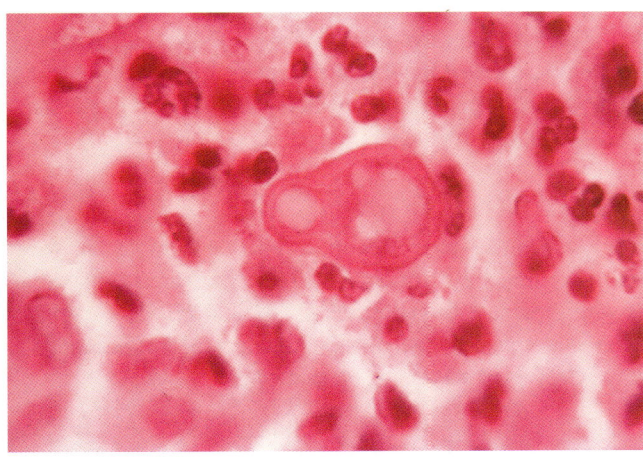

FIG. 9-10. Photomicrograph showing acute and chronic inflammation with microabscess and giant cells in blastomycosis.

TOXOPLASMOSIS

Presentation

Clinically, most patients with toxoplasmosis are in fact asymptomatic, although clinically overt disease may involve any organ system, including the central nervous system.

Pathophysiology

This infection is caused by *Toxoplasma gondii*, which is transmitted by ingestion of oocyst-containing cat feces or infected, poorly cooked lamb or pork.

Histology

The histologic appearance of a lymph node infected with toxoplasmosis is characteristic, with hyperplastic lymphoid follicles and germinal centers of variable size occupying the cortex. These may extend into the medullary cords of the node. Mitotic figures within germinal centers may be prominent, and macrophages containing bodies that can be tinged are often prominent and can be mistaken for the organism itself. Confirmation of the diagnosis of toxoplasmosis is only rarely accomplished by histologic identification of either the pseudocyst or true cyst in lymphoid tissue.

COCCIDIOIDOMYCOSIS

Presentation

Coccidioidomycosis is a fungal disease endemic to the southwestern United States and northern Mexico. It is spread by inhalation of spores, and the lungs are most commonly affected. Head and neck manifestations are rare but can involve the larynx to cause hoarseness or airway compromise.

Pathophysiology

The fungal disease can spread systemically and cause a granulomatous inflammatory reaction at any given site.

Histology

Histology often shows only formations of noncaseating granulomas with an inflammatory infiltrate. The diagnosis can be made only by using fungal stains to show the typical coccidioidal spherules filled with numerous endospores.

SARCOIDOSIS

Presentation

Sarcoidosis is a granulomatous disorder of unknown cause that may involve numerous systems. It commonly affects young adults, with the most frequent manifestation being that of bilateral hilar adenopathy combined with a pulmonary infiltrate and skin or eye lesions. There may be hypercalciuria with or without hypercalcemia.

Pathophysiology

The major manifestations of sarcoidosis fall into three categories: (1) chest radiographic abnormalities in an asymptomatic patient, (2) pulmonary symptoms, and (3) extrathoracic or systemic symptoms. The 20% of patients who present with systemic symptoms generally have fever, malaise, or weight loss with peripheral lymphadenopathy. Approximately 60% of patients with sarcoid granulomas will have elevated levels of serum angiotensin-converting enzyme.

Histology

The histologic appearance is that of noncaseating epithelioid cell granulomas in more than one organ. Langhans' giant cells may be present as well as intracytoplasmic inclusions, including calcified, laminated bodies (Schaumann's bodies).

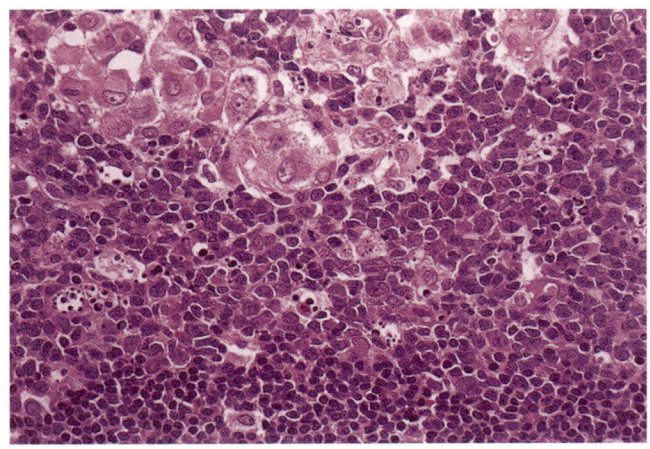

FIG. 9-11. Toxoplasmosis lymphadenitis.

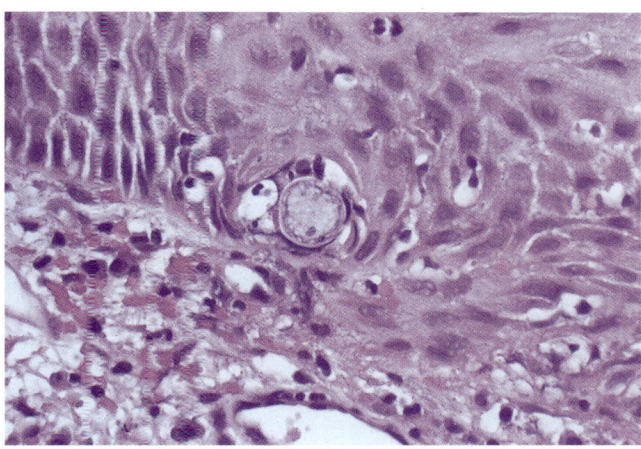

FIG. 9-12. Coccidioidomycosis of larynx.

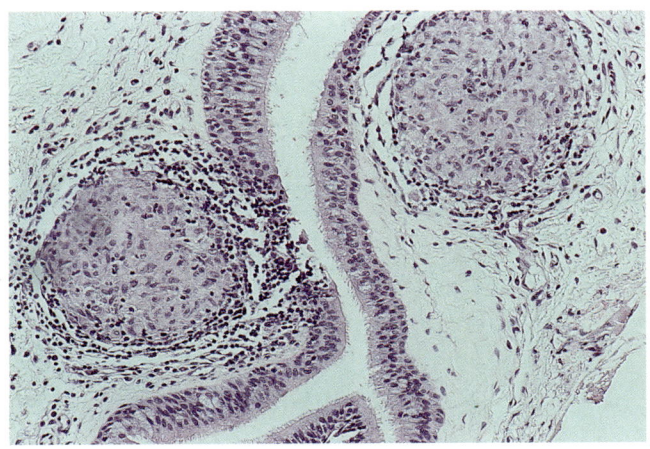

FIG. 9-13. Noncaseating granulomas of sarcoidosis in paranasal sinus stroma.

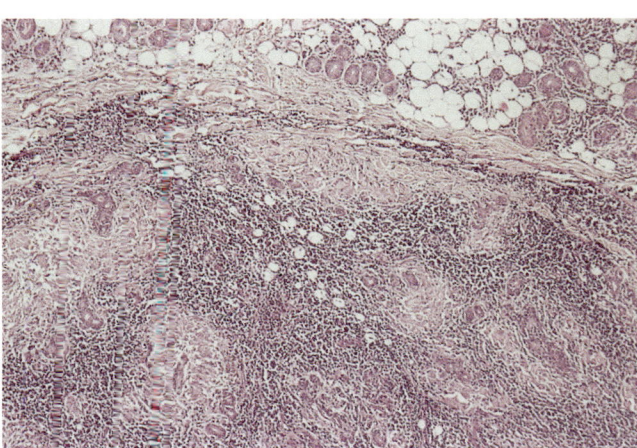

FIG. 9-14. Granulomatous (sarcoid) lymphadenitis in a parotid lymph node.

10

Benign Neoplasms

GRANULAR CELL TUMOR

Presentation

Granular cell tumors arise from Schwann cells. This tumor is frequently associated with an overlying pseudoepitheliomatous hyperplasia, which may lead to confusion with squamous cell carcinoma.

Pathophysiology

These lesions may occur anywhere in the head and neck but typically develop in the larynx or on the tongue.

Histology

Histologically, there is a poorly circumscribed lesion with a trabecular or nesting growth pattern composed of round cells that have a coarse, granular cytoplasm. A malignant granular cell tumor is very rare.

SCHWANNOMA AND NEUROFIBROMA

Presentation

Schwannomas usually present as an asymptomatic, slowly enlarging mass.

Pathophysiology

Schwannomas are benign tumors that arise from the Schwann cells of peripheral nerve sheaths. They may be found in any part of the body, but a significant minority occur in the head and neck. They are generally slow-growing tumors that are asymptomatic. A special type of schwannoma is the acoustic neuroma.

Histology

Histologically, the tumors contain regions of compact spindle cells known as Antoni A and loose hypocellular zones with peripheral palisading of cells known as Antoni B. Palisading nuclei aligned in rows are called Verocay bodies.

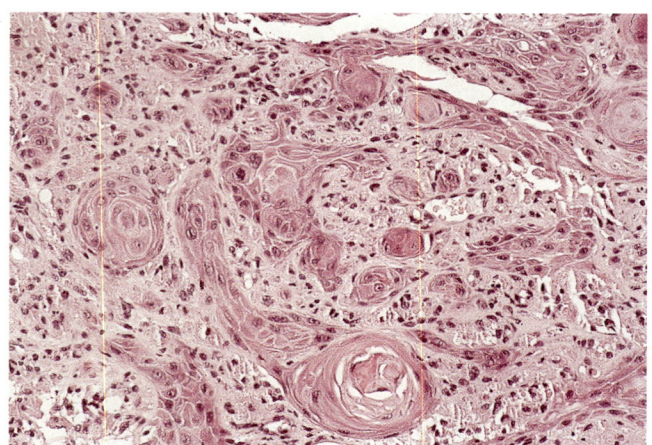 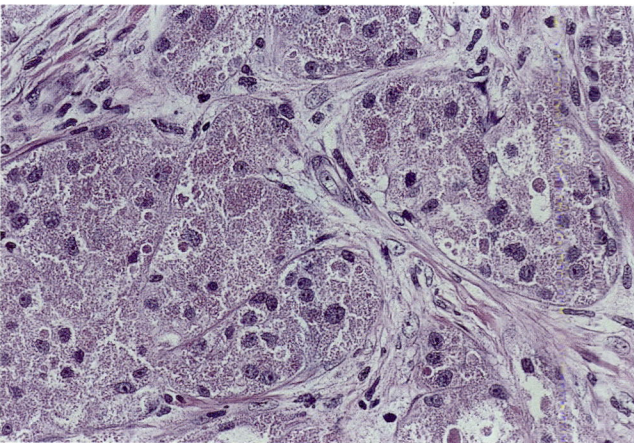

FIG. 10-1. A,B: Granular cell tumor in larynx. The pseudoepitheliomatous hyperplasia should not be mistaken for carcinoma.

Chapter 10/Benign Neoplasms

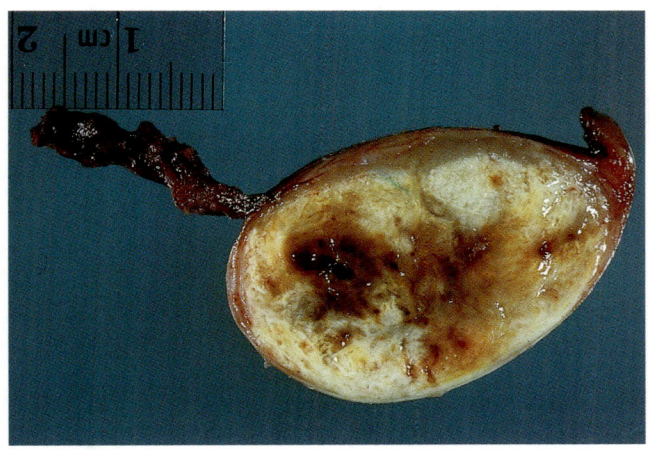

FIG. 10-2. So-called "ancient schwannoma" in neck.

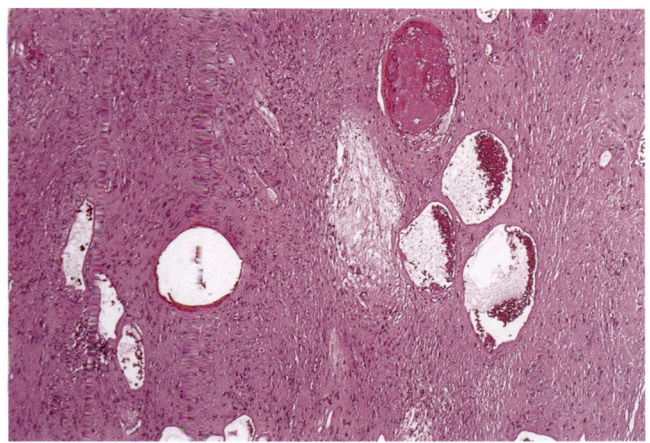

FIG. 10-3. Marked retrogressive changes in a schwannoma.

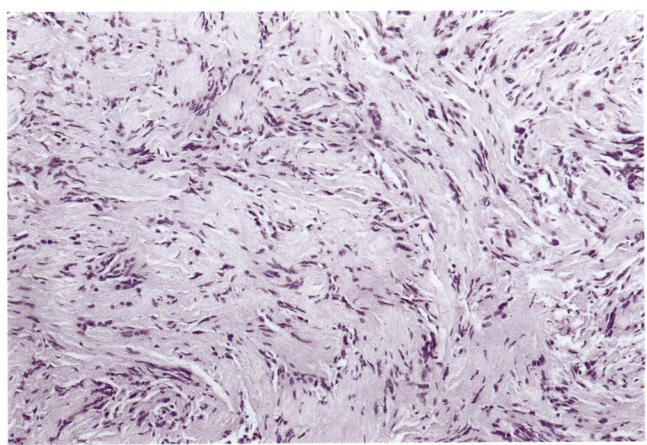

FIG. 10-4. Nasal schwannoma with Antoni A areas.

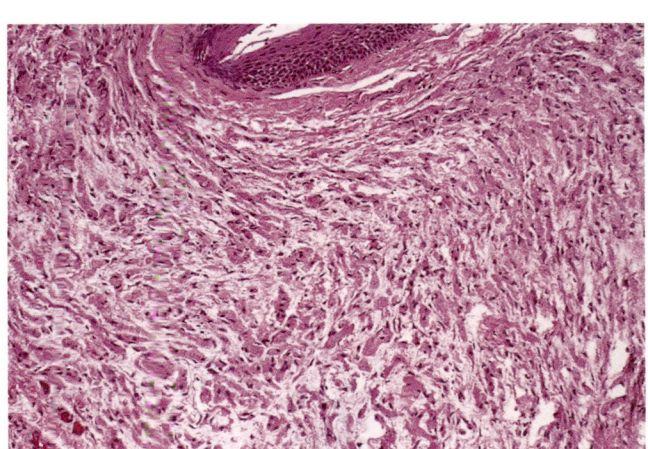

FIG. 10-5. Cutaneous neurofibroma.

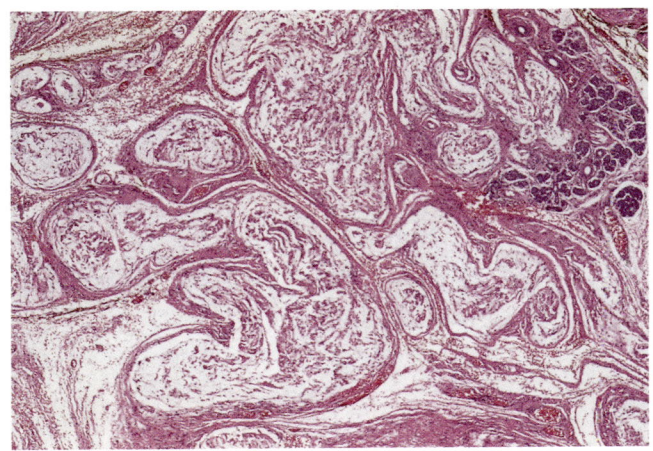
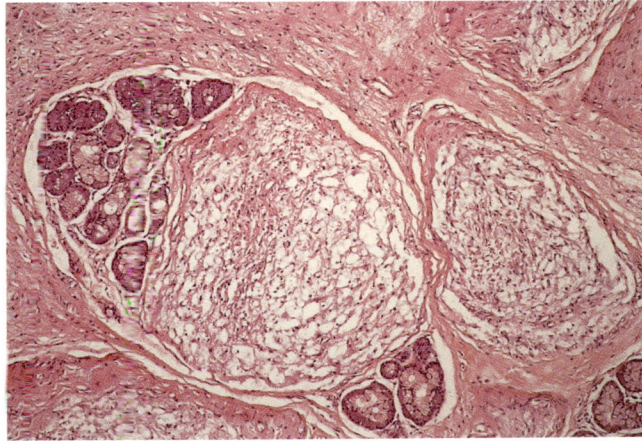

FIG. 10-6. A,B: Plexiform neurofibromas: of parotid gland in **A** and of larynx in **B**.

LIPOMA AND HIBERNOMA

Presentation

These tumors are generally solitary, slow-growing, well-circumscribed, asymptomatic, mobile masses.

Pathophysiology

Lipomas are benign, slow-growing tumors composed of mature fat cells. Approximately 23% occur in the head and neck.

Histology

Histologically, the tumor is composed of mature fat cells surrounded by a thin capsule. It is generally lobular.

RHABDOMYOMA

Presentation

Rhabdomyomas are slow-growing, asymptomatic masses.

Pathophysiology

Rhabdomyomas are rare benign tumors of skeletal muscle origin and are quite uncommon in the head and neck. There is an adult and an infantile form.

Histology

The adult tumors are composed of large, round cells with a granular, eosinophilic cytoplasm and peripheral nuclei. The infantile tumors, which are clearly different, are composed of spindled, elongated cells.

LEIOMYOMA

Presentation

These lesions typically present as a slowly enlarging asymptomatic mass. Pain is rarely part of the clinical picture. The tongue is the most common location in the head and neck, but fewer than 100 cases are reported in the literature. The rarity is not a consequence of histologic misdiagnosis but rather of the paucity of smooth muscle in this region.

Pathophysiology

It is felt that these tumors may originate from aberrant undifferentiated mesenchyme and/or smooth-muscle elements in the walls of blood vessels.

Histology

Leiomyomas are differentiated smooth-muscle tumors. The cells grow in winding bands or cords that tend to interlace. The nuclei are blunt-ended, and intracellular myofibrils can be found with ease. The nuclei tend to palisade. Marked vascularity is frequent.

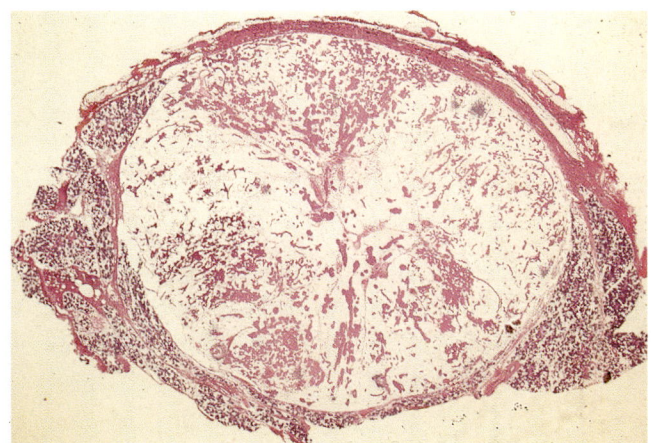

FIG. 10-7. Lipoma of parotid gland.

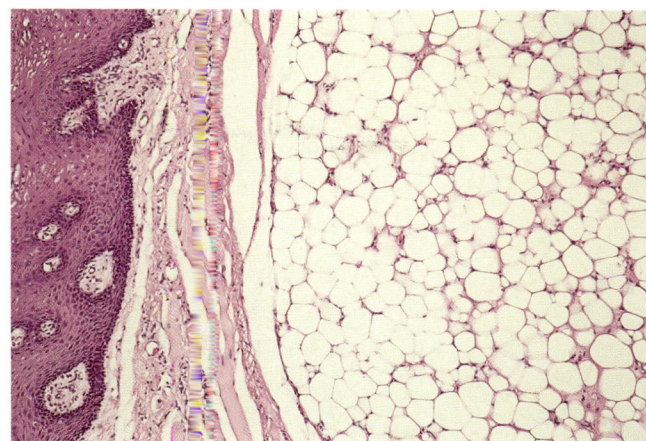

FIG. 10-8. Lipoma of tongue.

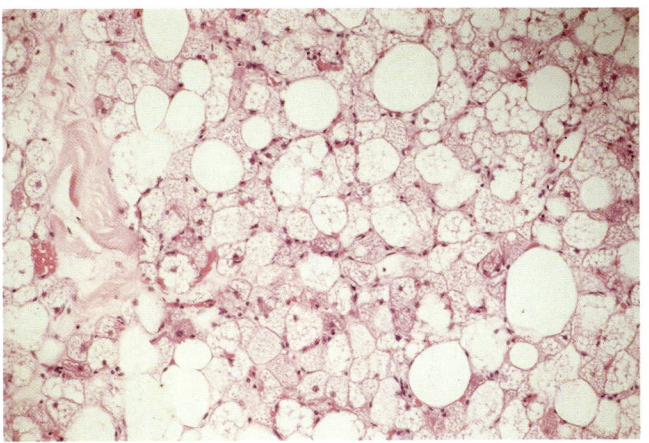

FIG. 10-9. Hibernoma.

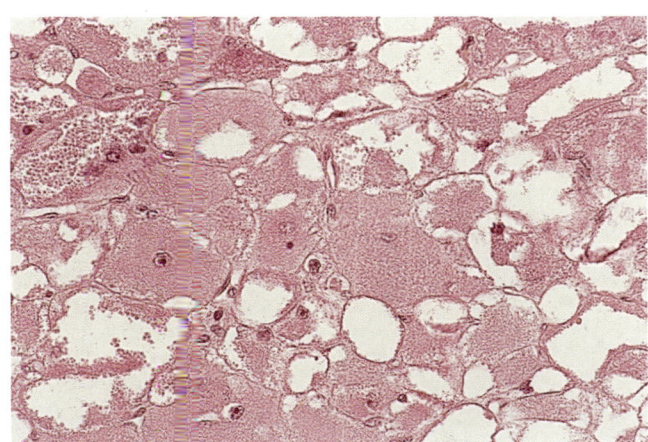

FIG. 10-10. Rhabdomyoma, adult type.

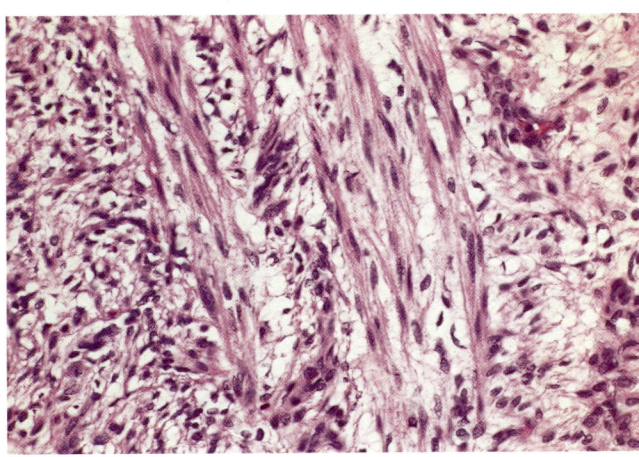

FIG. 10-11. Rhabdomyoma, infantile type.

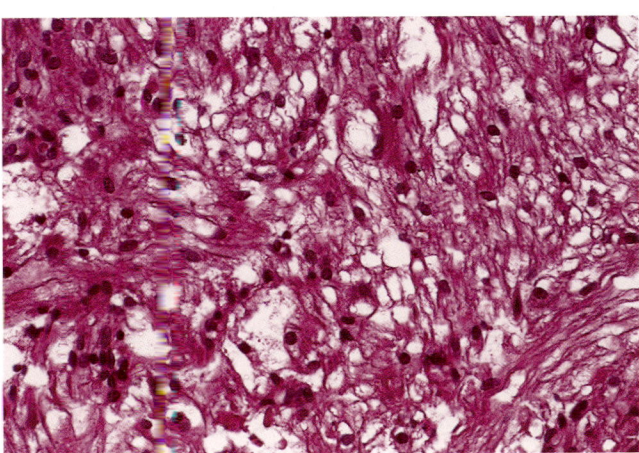

FIG 10-12. Leiomyoma in nasal cavity.

PARAGANGLIOMA

Presentation

Paragangliomas of the head and neck generally present as asymptomatic enlarging masses, except for those in the temporal bone, which affect hearing.

Pathophysiology

These tumors arise from neural crest cells and generally occur in three locations in the head and neck—the carotid body, vagus nerve, and jugular foramen, although other sites may be affected. The benign tumors are usually slowly progressive. A small number are malignant.

Histology

The usual appearance is that of an organoid neoplasm, composed of epithelioid cells divided and surrounded by a richly vascular stroma. The alveolar cells are usually closely packed. The cytoplasm is typically abundant, clear, and pale-staining or finely granular and eosinophilic. Mitotic figures are rare.

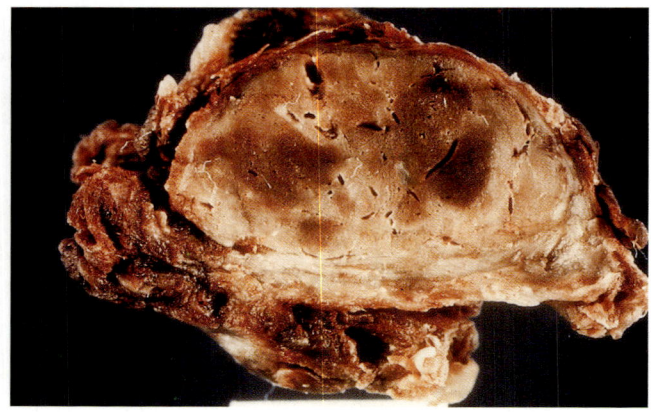

FIG. 10-13. Carotid body paraganglioma.

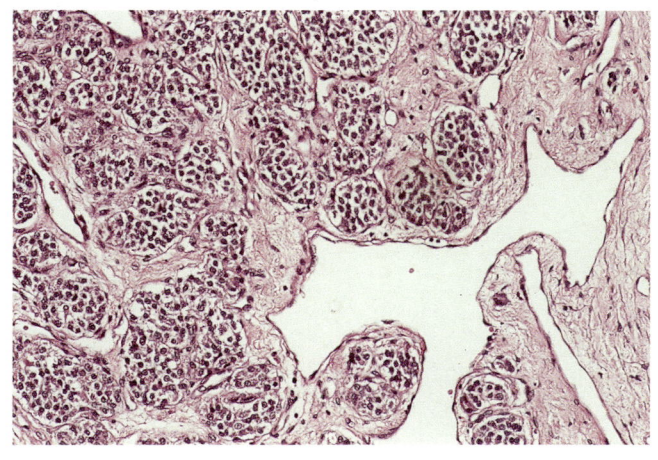
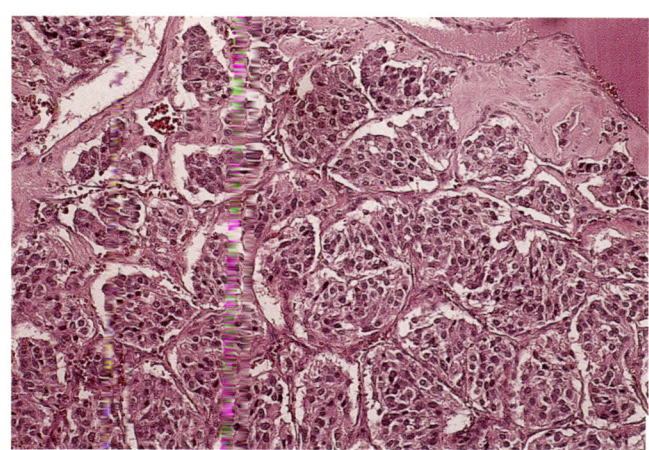
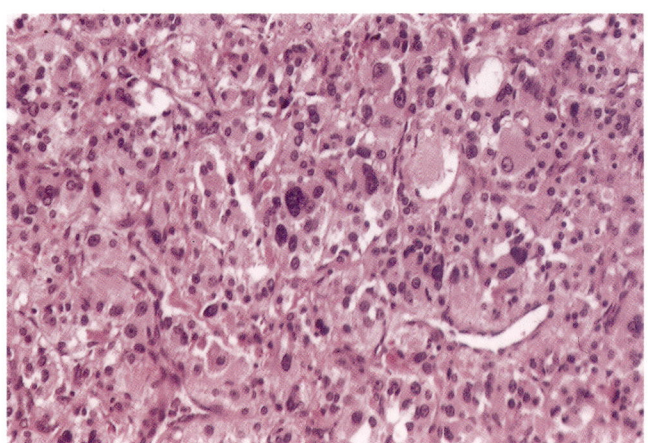

FIG. 10-14. A–C: Carotid body paraganglioma. Zellballen aggregates of chief and sustentacular cells.

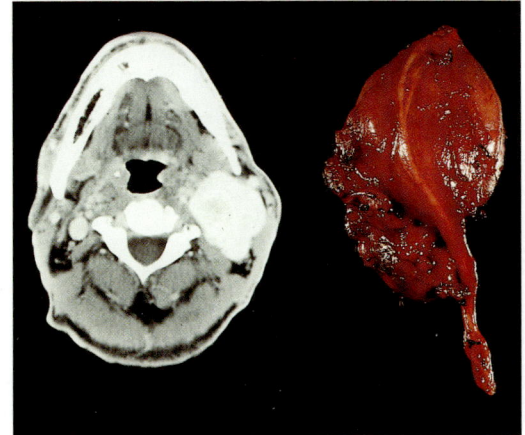
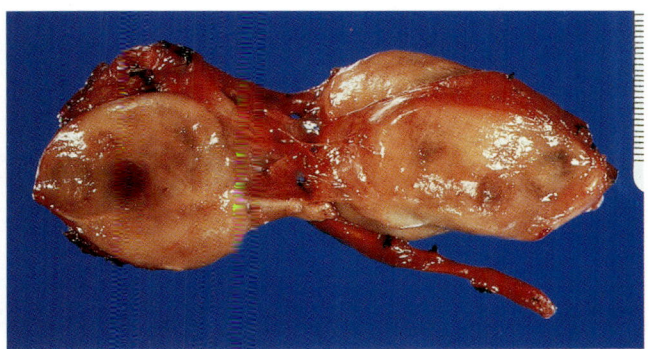

FIG. 10-15. A,B: Vagal body paraganglioma.

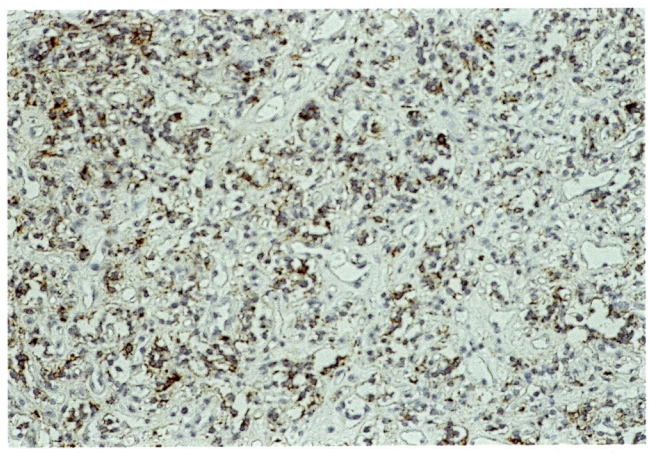

FIG. 10-16. Carotid body paraganglioma stained to demonstrate the chromogranin content in the chief cells.

11

Malignant Neoplasms

SQUAMOUS CELL CARCINOMA

Presentation

Squamous cell carcinoma of the mucous membranes is the most common tumor of the head and neck. The early appearance of these neoplasms may be quite variable, and the possibility of an early diagnosis is often site-dependent. The very earliest manifestation of these lesions is probably erythroplakia, which is a clinical term describing an area of mucous membrane that is redder than normal. A very high percentage of biopsy specimens, up to 91%, from erythroplakic lesions show invasive carcinoma, carcinoma *in situ*, or severe dysplasia. Another appearance is termed leukoplakia, which is a whitish appearance to the mucous membrane. Any lesion that causes a thickening in the mucous membrane will have a white appearance, as it masks the underlying blood supply, which is the reason for the pink-to-red appearance. However, the term is used clinically. When biopsy specimens are taken, the lesion may show nothing more than hyperkeratosis. On the other hand, the tissue may also show varying degrees of dysplasia or even invasive carcinoma.

Pathophysiology

It is likely that squamous carcinomas of the upper aerodigestive tract undergo the same histopathologic changes over time as those of the uterine cervix, with progressive dysplasia leading to carcinoma *in situ* and finally to invasive carcinoma. Carcinoma *in situ* (intraepithelial carcinoma) is a microscopic, not a clinical, diagnosis, and the term is used to describe severe dysplasia that may involve the entire epithelium from the basement membrane to the epithelial surface.

In general terms, squamous cell carcinoma accounts for 70% to 90% of all carcinomas of the mucous membranes in the head and neck. These carcinomas occur more commonly in men than in women and usually can be associated with alcohol and tobacco consumption. The risk for some cancers is as much as 15 times greater in persons who are heavy users of alcohol and tobacco than in those who use neither.

Histology

Classically, squamous cell carcinoma shows nests and cords of epithelial cells with varying degrees of penetration of the subepithelial structures. In reality, however, great variation is possible, as the figures show.

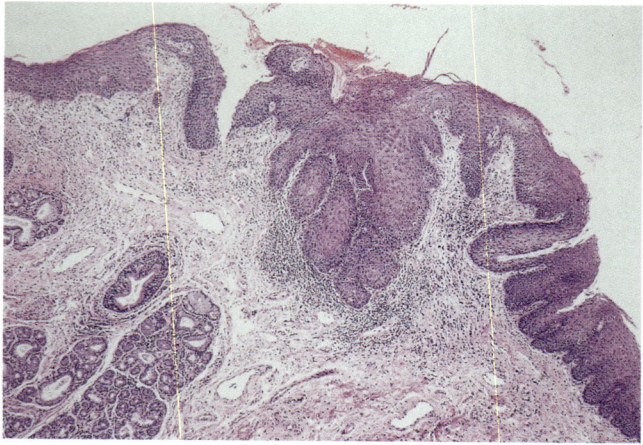

FIG. 11-1. A microcarcinoma (of supraglottis, well-differentiated invasive squamous cell carcinoma).

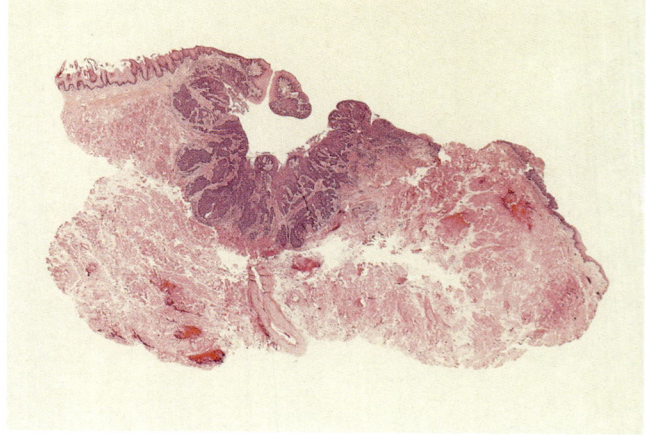

FIG. 11-2. Deeply invasive squamous cell carcinoma of tongue.

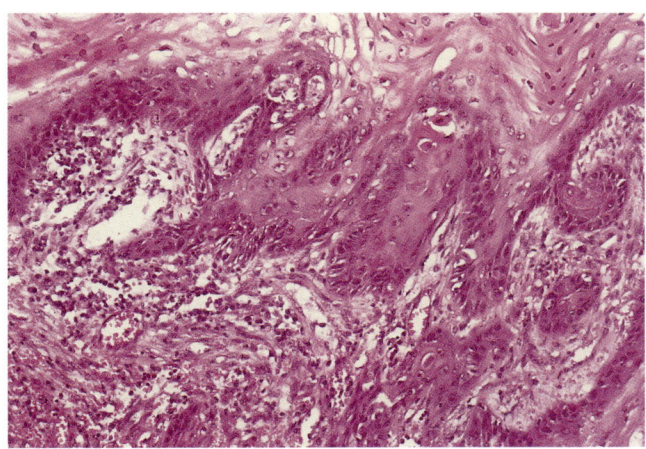

FIG. 11-3. Invasive, well-differentiated squamous cell carcinoma of oral cavity.

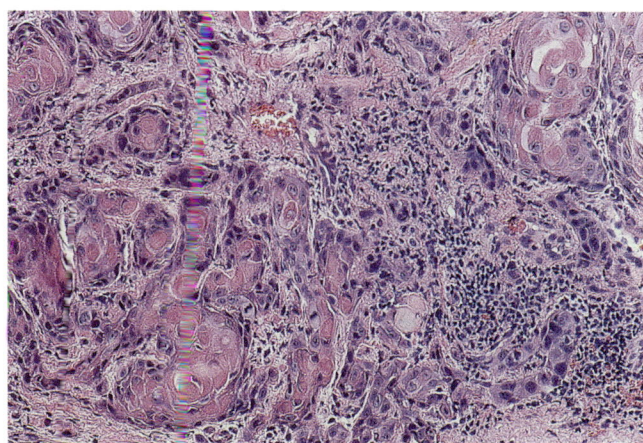

FIG. 11-4. Invasive, well-differentiated squamous cell carcinoma of oral cavity. Note the difference in mode of invasion from the carcinoma in Fig. 11-3.

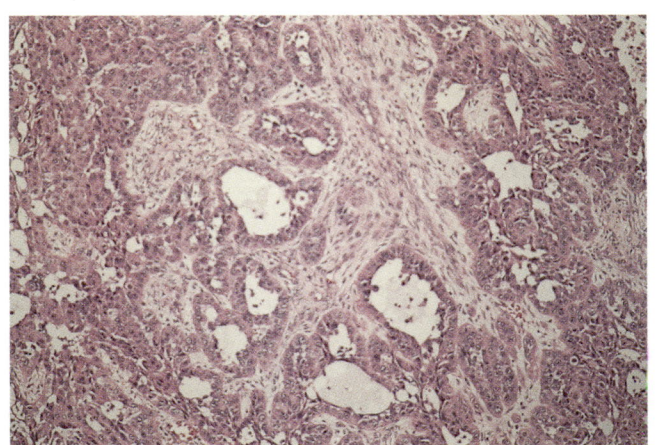
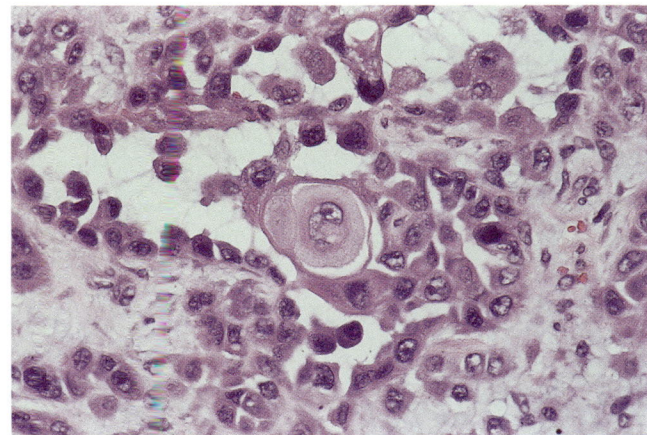

FIG. 11-5. A,B: Adenoid squamous cell carcinoma of pharynx. The glandlike (adenoid) pattern is brought about by acantholysis, seen well in **B**.

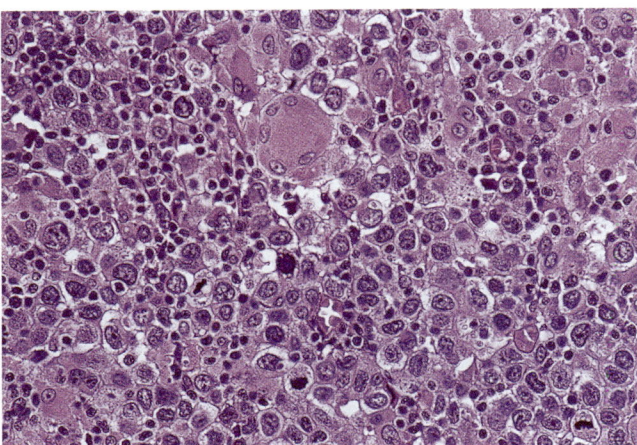

FIG. 11-6. Poorly differentiated squamous cell carcinoma.

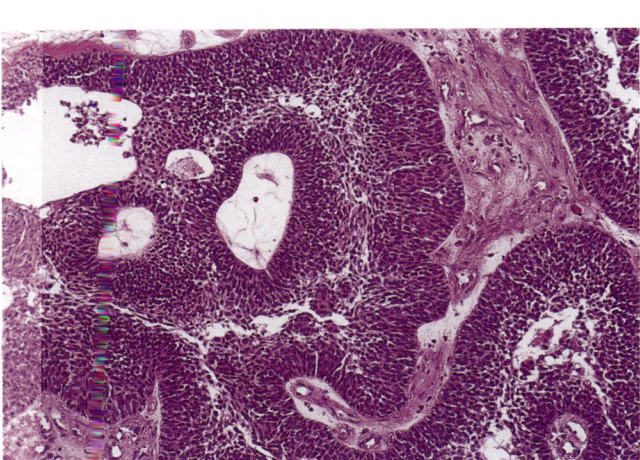

FIG. 11-7. Nonkeratinizing squamous cell carcinoma of tonsil.

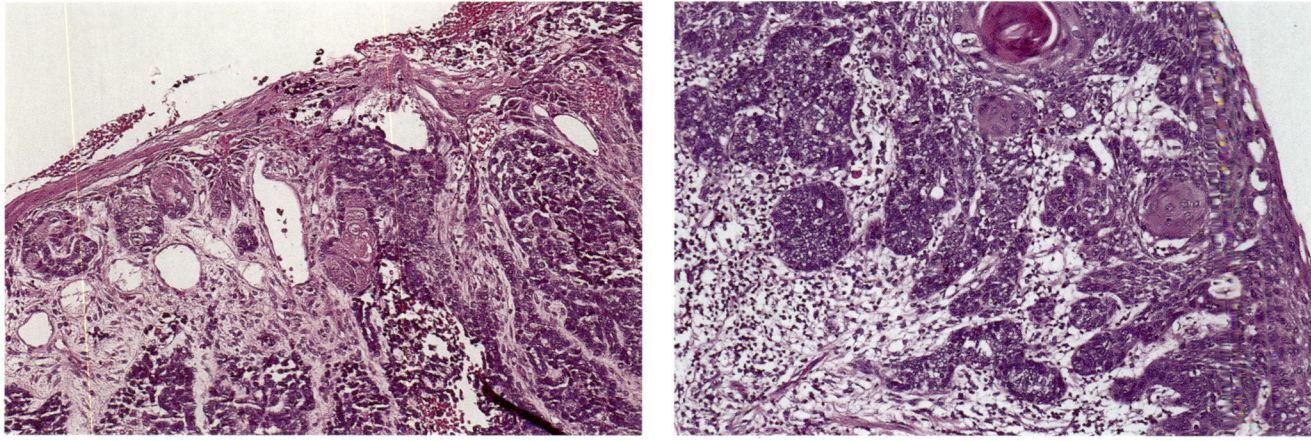

FIG. 11-8. A,B: Basaloid squamous cell carcinoma of oropharynx. In this example, origin from the surface mucosa is seen. Moreover, there is a combination of definable squamous carcinoma and the basaloid component.

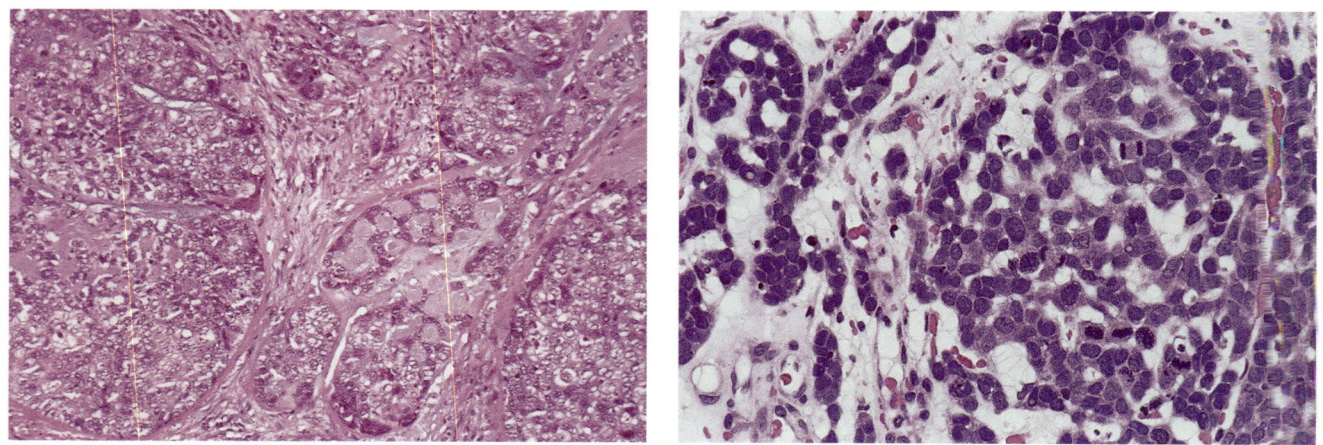

FIG. 11-9. A,B: Basaloid squamous cell carcinoma with adenoid cystic carcinoma-like features.

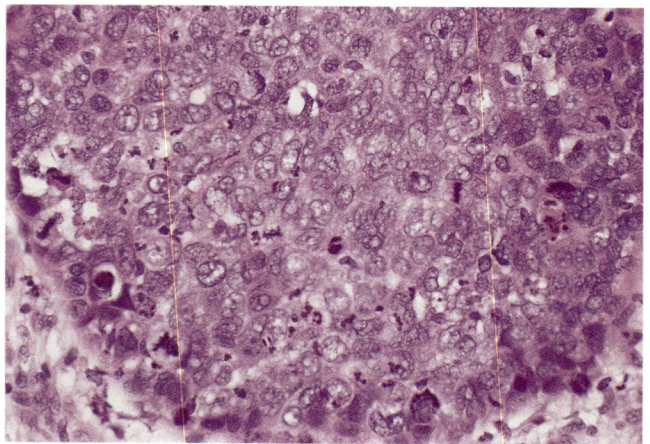

FIG. 11-10. The high-grade histologic feature of basaloid squamous cell carcinoma is clear in this undifferentiated area.

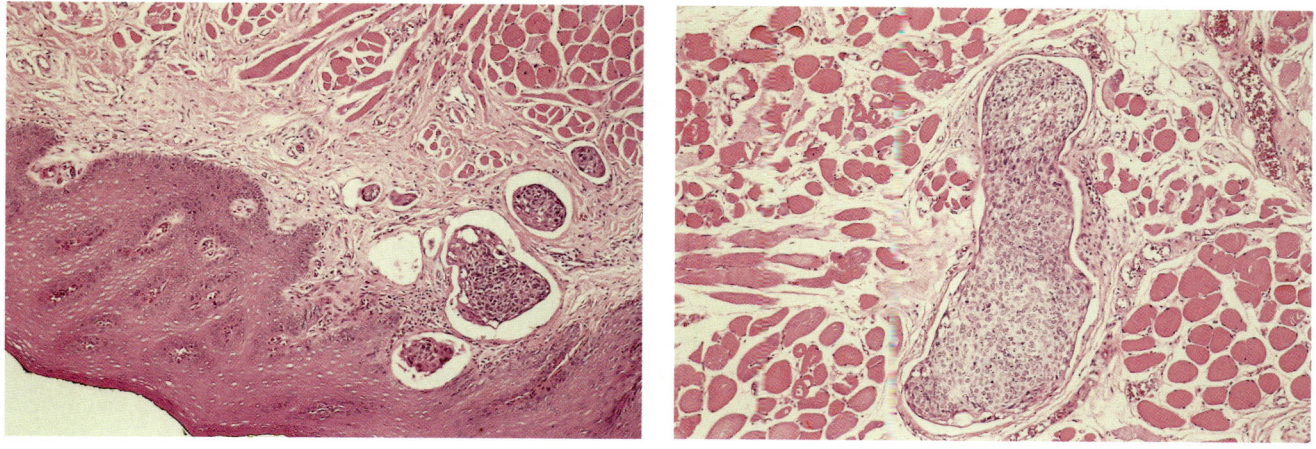

FIG. 11-11. A,B: Submucosal lymphatics containing squamous cell tumor emboli.

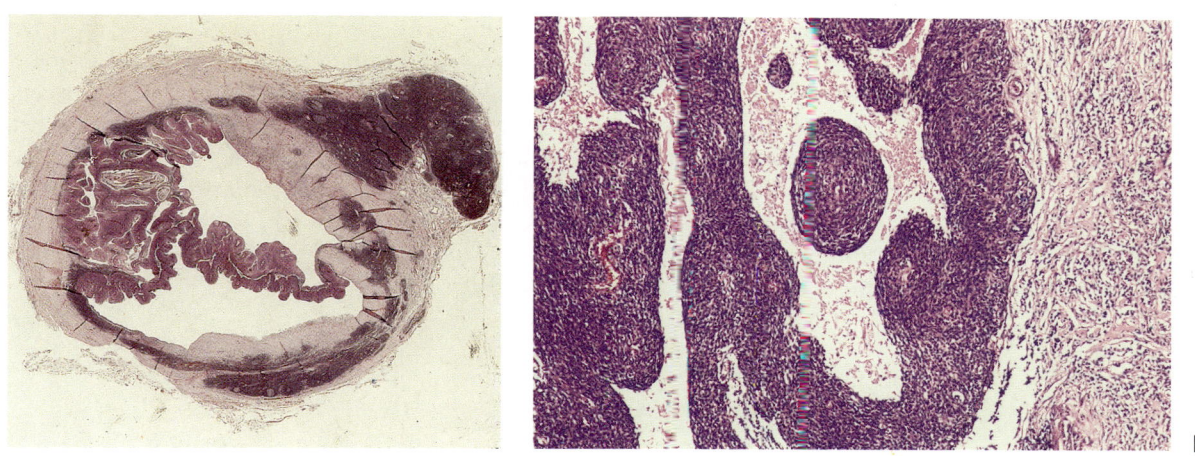

FIG. 11-12. A,B: Cystic metastatic squamous cell carcinoma in cervical lymph node. Although not pathognomonic, this cystic architecture strongly suggests a primary tumor in the ipsilateral tonsil.

SQUAMOUS CELL CARCINOMA VARIANTS

Squamous cell carcinoma is not a homogeneous entity. It has several phenotypic expressions: keratinizing and nonkeratinizing, papillary or verrucous, and nonverrucous (exophytic or endophytic), basaloid, and sarcomatoid. Each has a univariate prognostic significance, along with the level of differentiation (well, moderately, poorly differentiated). Thickness of the carcinoma and depth of invasion, and especially size and clinical stage, are far more important and reliable predictors of clinical aggressiveness. Metastasis to cervical lymph nodes is an ominous prognostic sign that is accentuated when transcapsular extension of the metastasis into soft tissue is present.

A distinction must be made between verrucous carcinoma and conventional, well-differentiated squamous cell carcinoma. The former is an extremely well-differentiated carcinoma without metastatic potential but capable of significant local invasion.

Histologic variants tend to occur in certain sites: basaloid squamous cell carcinoma in the supraglottic larynx and oropharynx, nonkeratinizing squamous cell carcinoma in the nasopharynx and Waldeyer's ring epithelium, and verrucous carcinoma in the oral cavity and glottic and supraglottic larynx.

Obtaining an accurate histologic diagnosis of sarcomatoid (metaplastic) squamous cell carcinoma can be equally difficult and frustrating. Definable carcinoma may be elusive and small in the usually polypoid lesion. Epithelial malignancy ranges from carcinoma *in situ* to deeply invasive carcinoma and from well differentiated to poorly differentiated. It is the sarcoma-like component, however, that gives the carcinoma its name. Now believed to be a divergent differentiation of squamous cell carcinoma, sarcomatoid carcinoma can be obviously malignant (even simulating malignant fibrous histiocytoma) or deceptively innocuous in appearance. Diagnostic aid is provided by immunohistochemical detection of cytokeratin antigens in the sarcomatoid cells. This technique is not infallible, as up to 15% of sarcomatoid carcinomas do not demonstrate positive immunoreactivity, and some reactive myofibroblastic proliferations show a cross-reactivity to keratin antibodies. Consideration must also be given to the true pseudosarcomatous polypoid reaction to injury characterized by myofibroblastic proliferation.

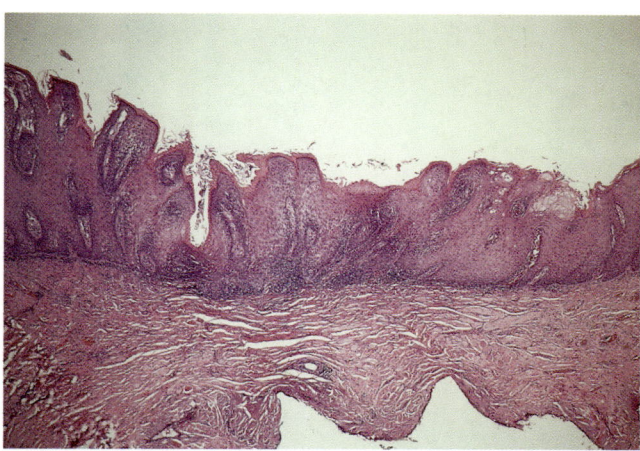

FIG. 11-13. Verrucous hyperplasia of oral mucosa. This forerunner of verrucous carcinoma displays nearly all the clinical behavior of verrucous carcinoma.

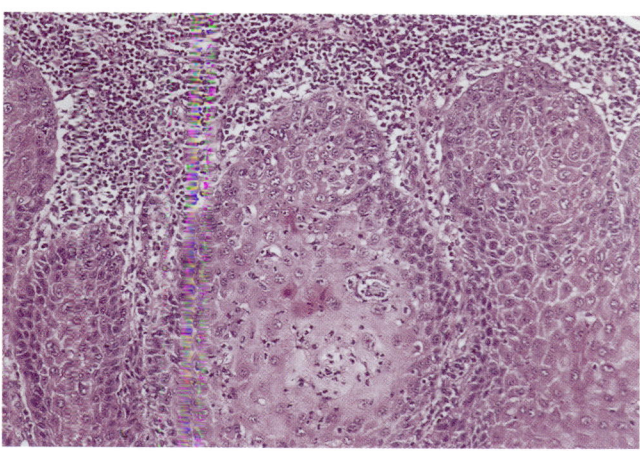

FIG. 11-14. Verrucous carcinoma. The blunt invasion of the carcinoma is often accompanied by a chronic inflammatory cell infiltrate.

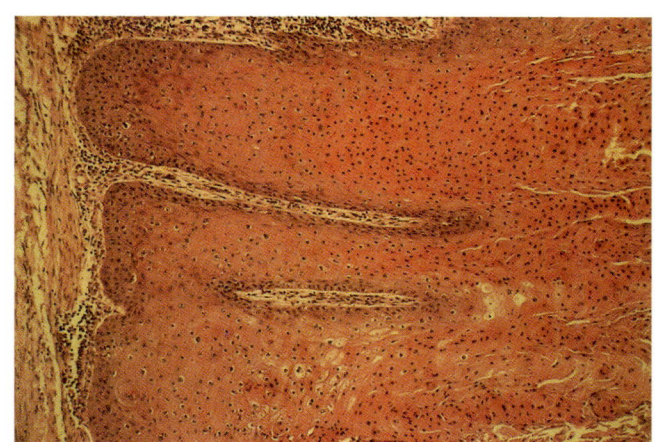

FIG. 11-15. Verrucous carcinoma showing a "regimented" morphology.

A B

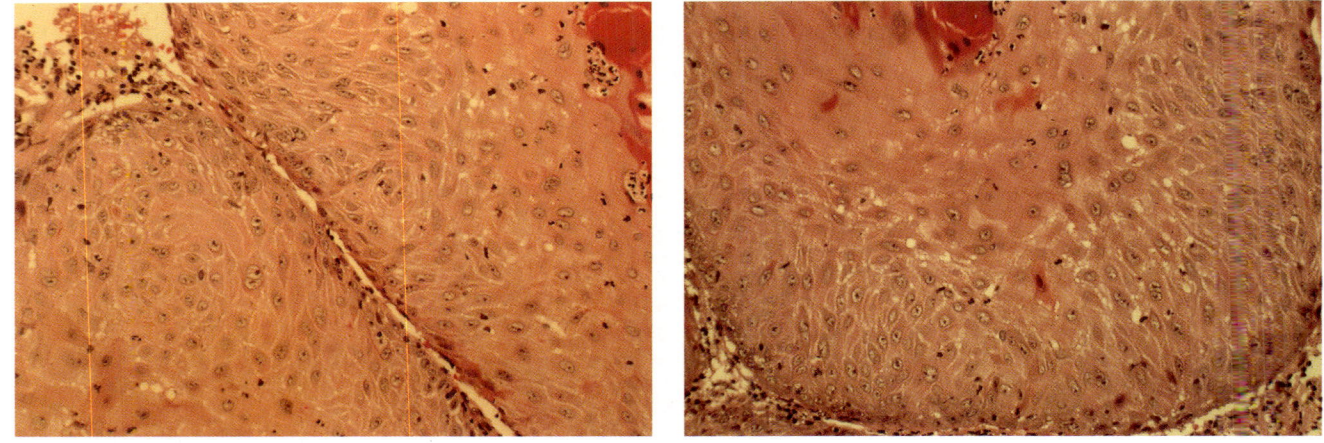

FIG. 11-16. A,B: Verrucous carcinoma in the deep invasive zone.

A B C

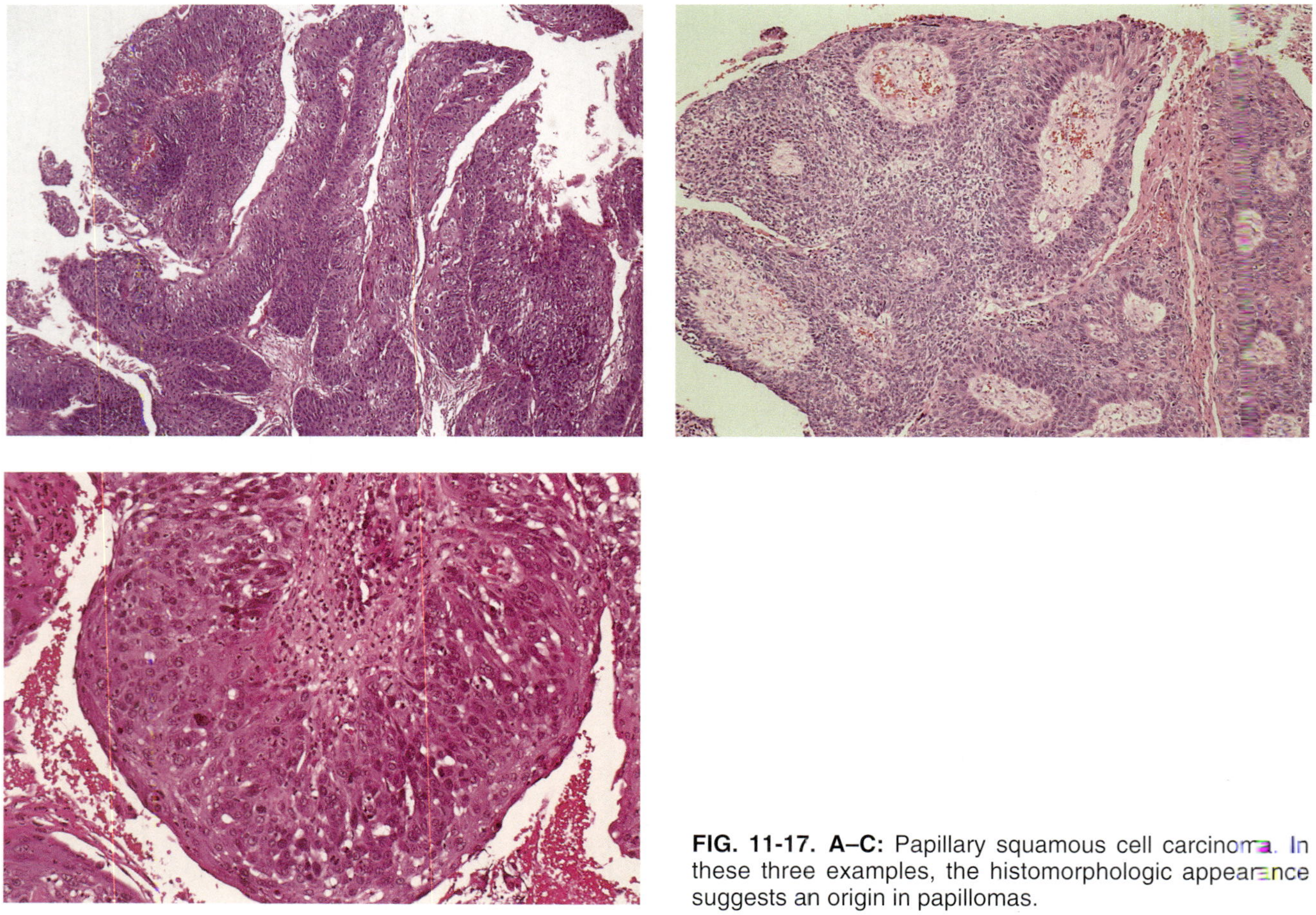

FIG. 11-17. A–C: Papillary squamous cell carcinoma. In these three examples, the histomorphologic appearance suggests an origin in papillomas.

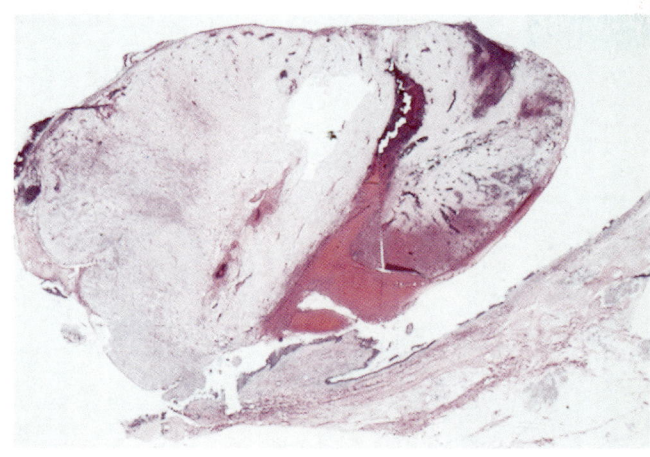 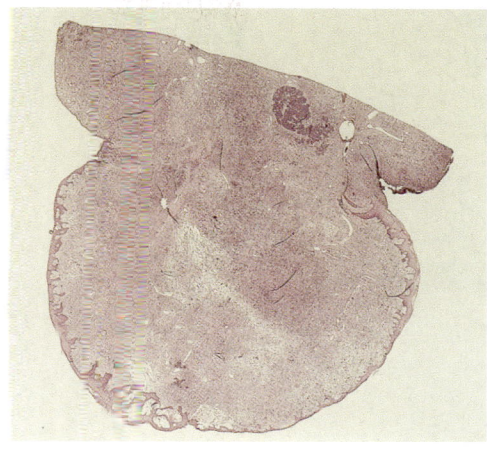

FIG. 11-18. A, B: Polypoid configuration of sarcomatoid carcinoma. The specimen in **A** is from the larynx, and there is no discernible squamous carcinoma. The specimen in **B** is from the oral cavity, and areas of squamous cell carcinoma persist.

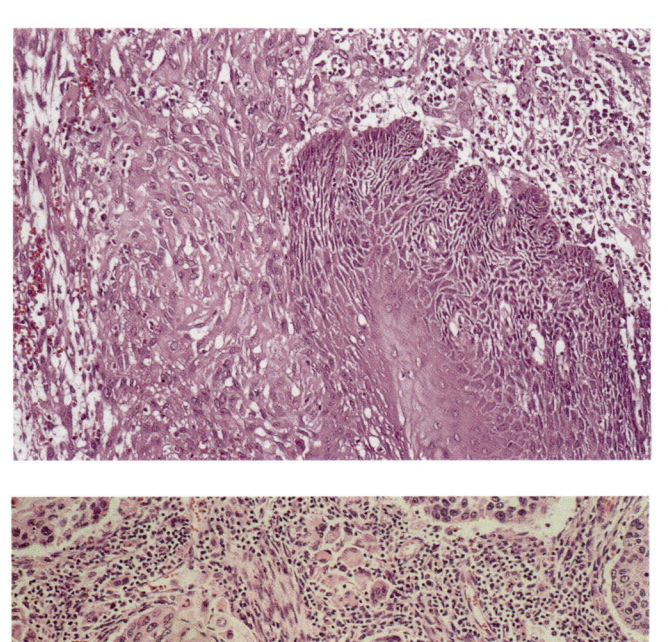 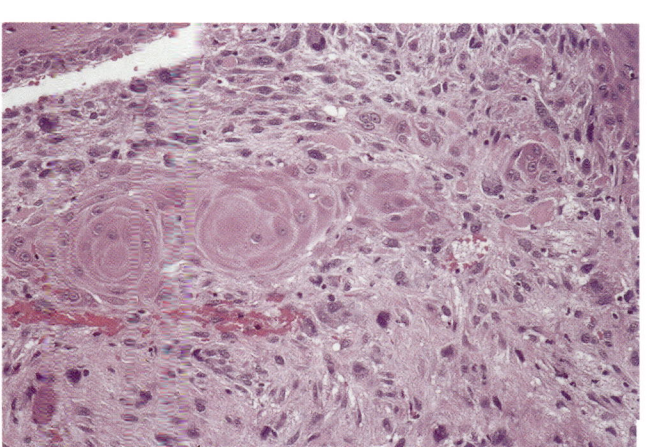

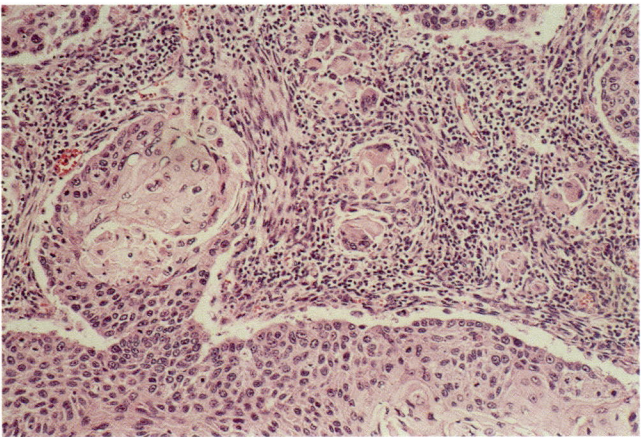

FIG. 11-19 A–C: Sarcomatoid carcinoma. In each of these examples, there is a definable and easily recognized squamous cell carcinoma.

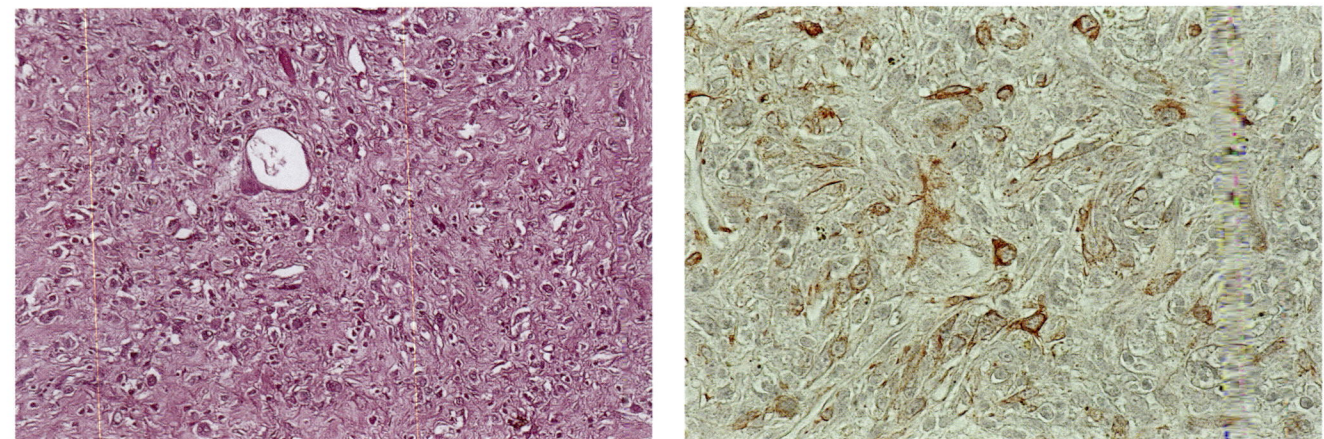

FIG. 11-20. A,B: Sarcomatoid carcinoma. The positive immunoreaction for cytokeratin in the neoplastic cells in **B** removes diagnostic doubt.

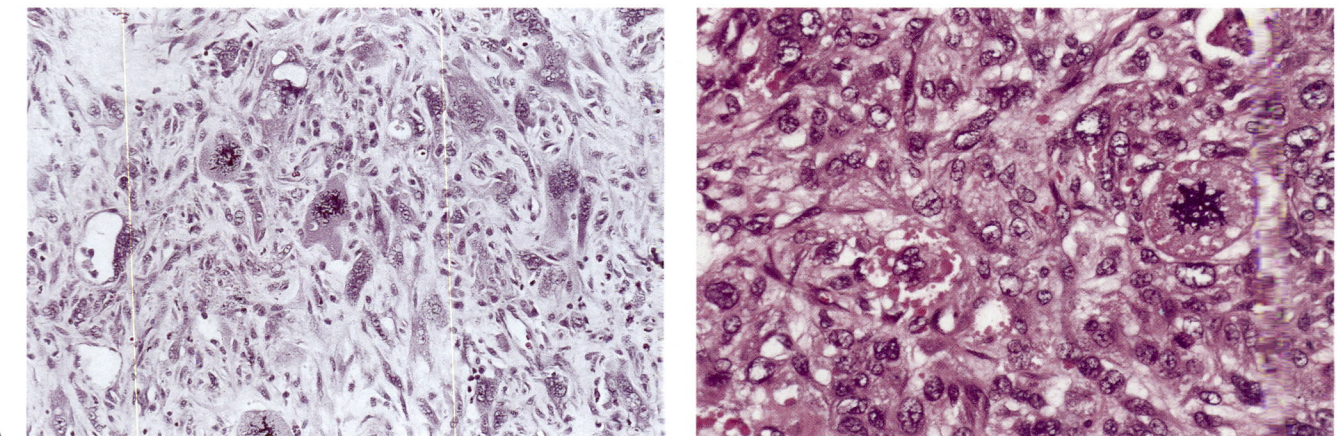

FIG. 11-21. A,B: Bizarre mitotic figures in a sarcomatoid carcinoma.

Chapter 11/Malignant Neoplasms 155

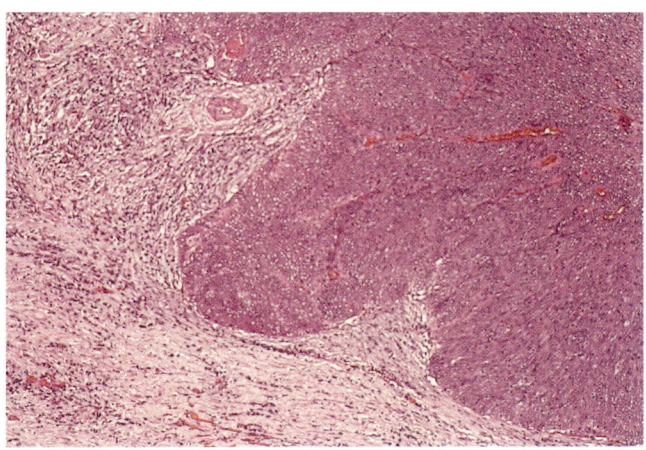

FIG. 11-22. Lymph node with extracapsular extension of metastasis.

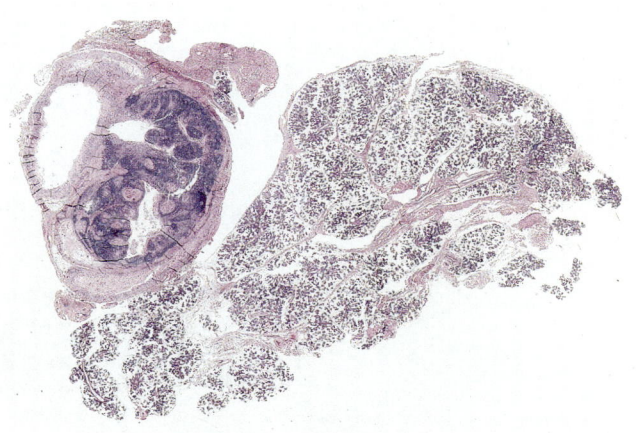

FIG. 11-23. Solitary intranodal metastasis in parotid lymph node.

RHABDOMYOSARCOMA

Presentation

These tumors usually present as rapidly enlarging masses in children under the age of 10 years.

Pathophysiology

Rhabdomyosarcoma is a malignant tumor of mesenchyme that occurs most commonly in children and young adults. It is the most common sarcoma of the head and neck and develops in a variety of locations. Survival is related to stage, with a progressive decrease in survival noted from stage I to stage IV.

Histology

Histologically, there are four variants: embryonal, alveolar, pleomorphic, and mixed. The embryonal variant consists of both round and spindle cells. The alveolar variant consists of noncohesive cells with central areas that are hypocellular, giving the appearance of alveoli. The pleomorphic variant is composed of pleomorphic cells admixed with spindle-shaped cells, whereas the mixed variant is composed of two or more histologic types.

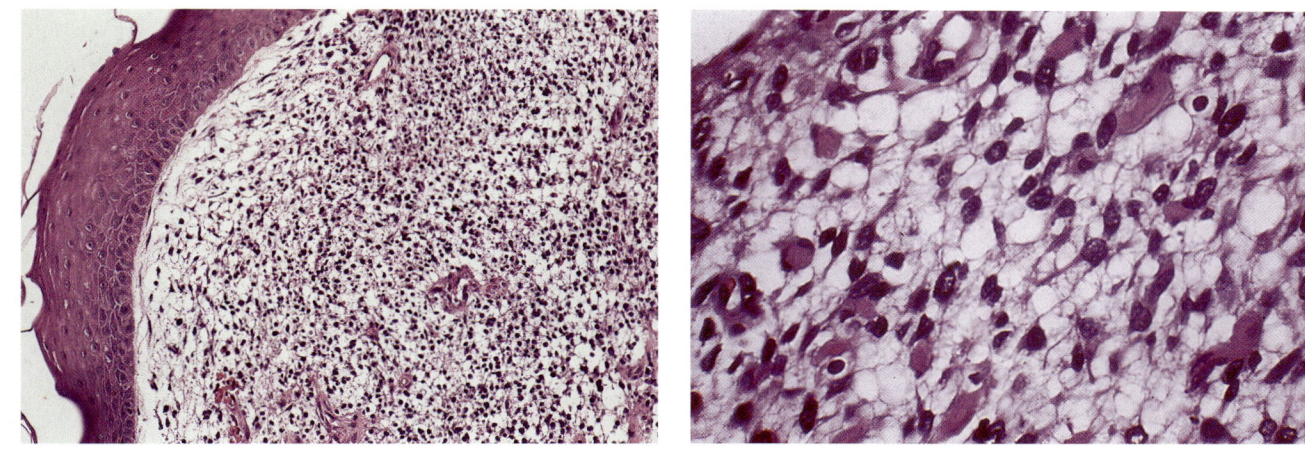

FIG. 11-24. A,B: Embryonal rhabdomyosarcoma, sinonasal tract.

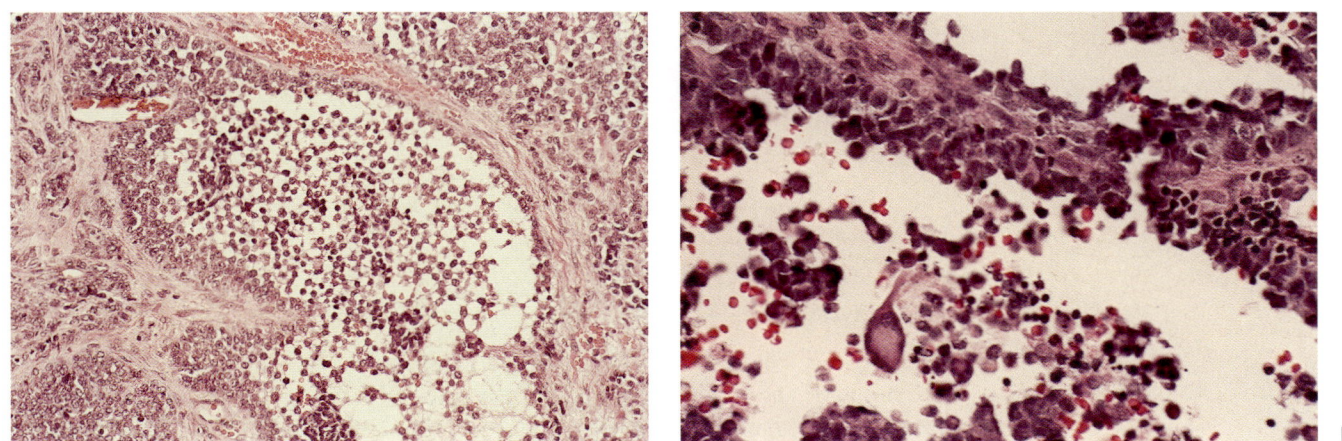

FIG. 11-25. A,B: Alveolar rhabdomyosarcoma.

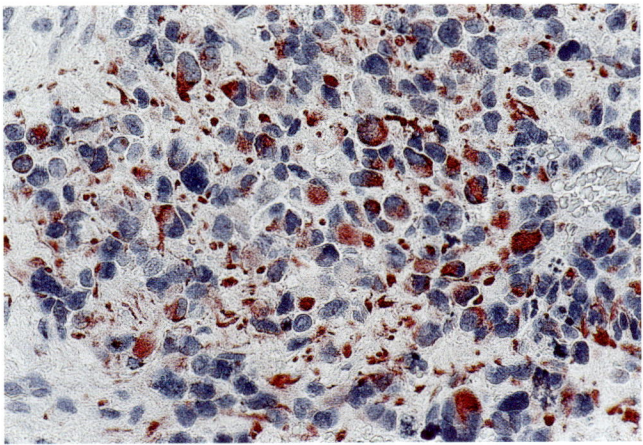

FIG. 11-26. Rhabdomyosarcoma of paranasal sinus showing antidesmin immunoreactivity.

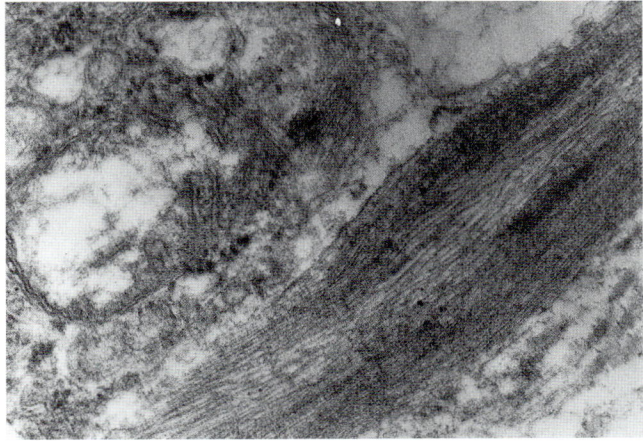

FIG. 11-27. Electron-optic micrograph of a rhabdomyosarcoma showing typical filaments.

LYMPHOMA

Presentation

Primary lymphomas of the head and neck may be of any histologic type, but they are generally non-Hodgkin's lymphomas. The presentation is that of an enlarging mass. The treatment depends on the histologic type as well as the stage.

Pathophysiology

As elsewhere in the body, lymphomas in the head and neck are nodal, extranodal, or both. The sinonasal tract is the location of most extranodal lymphomas (B- or T-cell), with prognosis dependent on stage and grade of the lymphoma. Compared with Wegener's granulomatosis, midfacial lymphomas are much more destructive of tissue. The majority of lymphomas afflicting the parotid glands are nodal. Sjögren's syndrome may precede either nodal or extranodal (salivary parenchymal) lymphomas.

Histology

The histologic appearance depends on the cell type; the working formulation classification is most commonly used.

PLASMACYTOMA

Presentation

The presentation is site-dependent, but the tumor usually presents as an asymptomatic, enlarging mass.

Pathophysiology

The plasma cell disorders comprise multiple myeloma, plasma cell leukemia, solitary plasmacytoma of bone, and extramedullary plasmacytoma. The most common region of involvement for extramedullary plasmacytoma is the head and neck (pharynx, nasopharynx, larynx, and oral cavity). Recurrences are common, and there is always the possibility of evolution to multiple myeloma or myelomatosis.

Histology

Most often a submucosal polyp, extramedullary plasmacytoma is usually solitary and composed of a pure culture of plasma cells. Amyloid may be occasionally seen in association with the plasmacytoma.

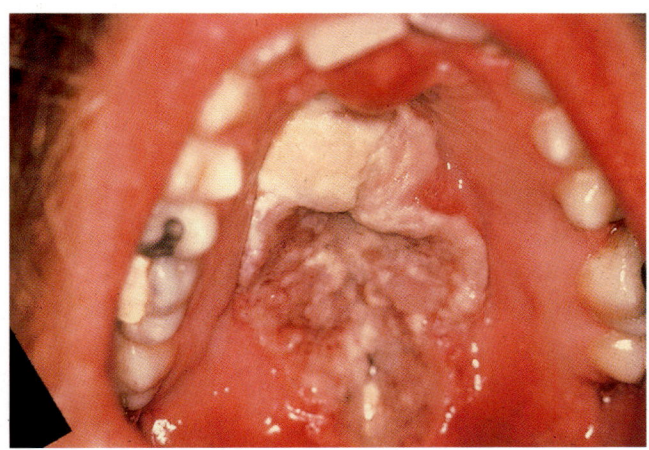

FIG. 11-28. Extensive palatal ulcer in a patient with paranasal sinus B-cell (high-grade) lymphoma.

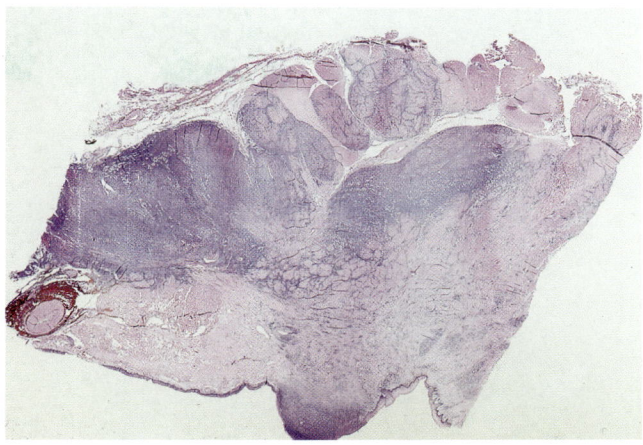

FIG. 11-29. Non-Hodgkin's B-cell lymphoma arising in base of tongue.

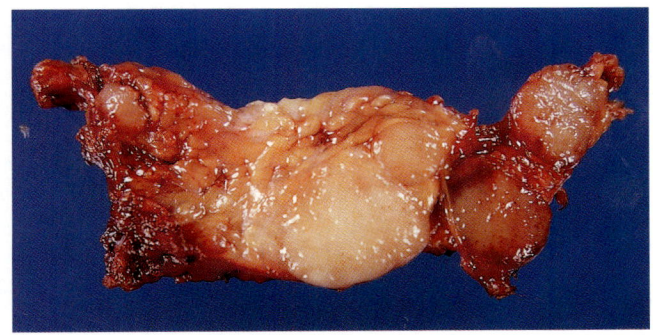

FIG. 11-30. Non-Hodgkin's lymphoma involving parotid gland.

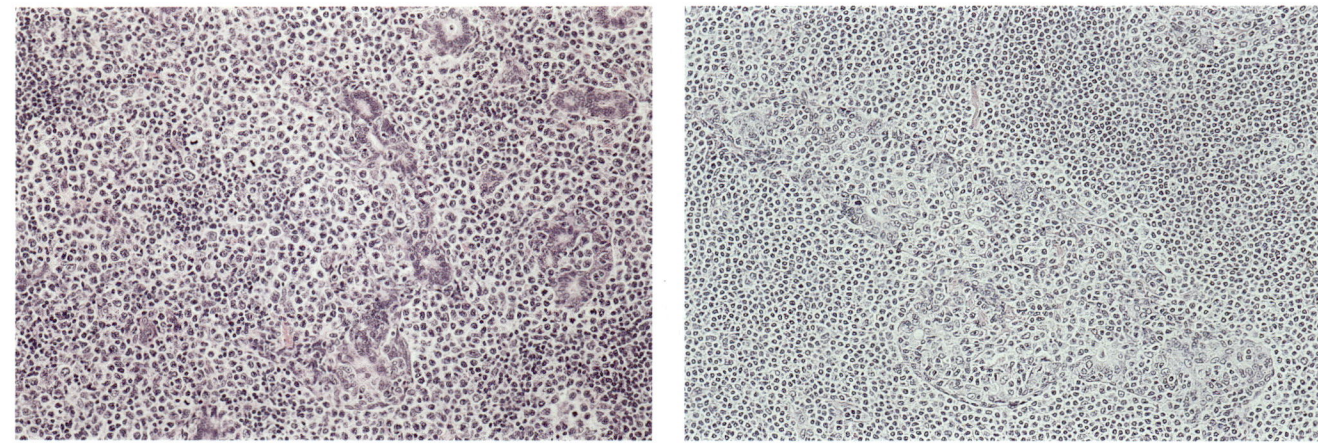

FIG. 11-31. A,B: B-cell lymphoma of mucosa-associated lymphoid tissue (MALT) origin from a patient with clinical Sjögren's syndrome.

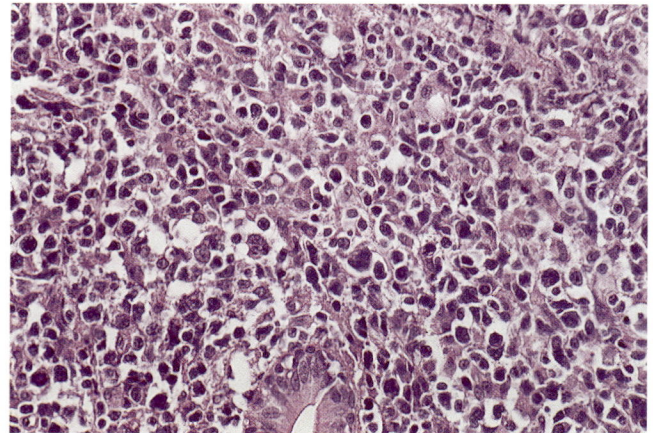

FIG. 11-32. High-grade diffuse lymphoma in the sinonasal tract.

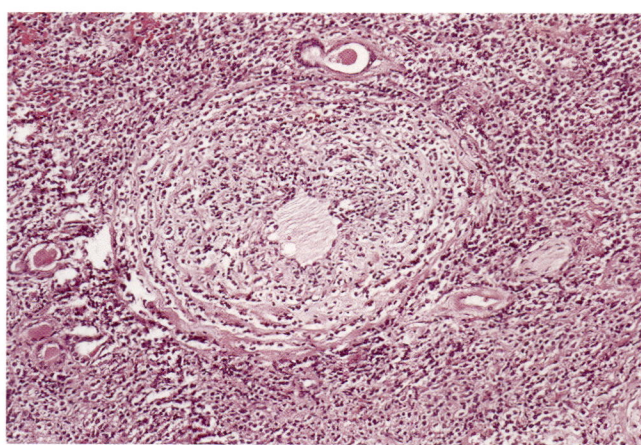

FIG. 11-33. Nasal lymphoma showing prominent angiocentrism.

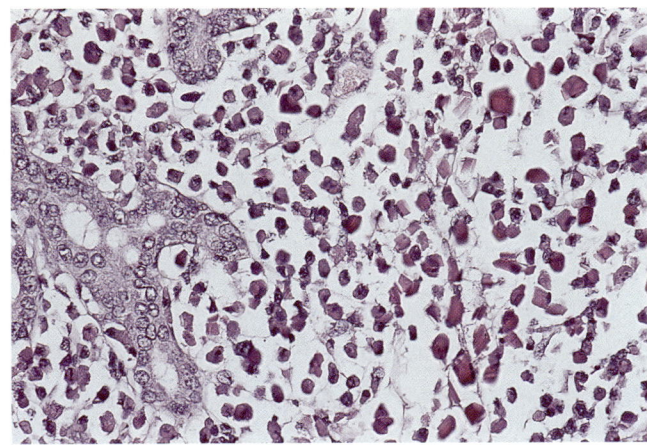

FIG. 11-34. A so-called "immunocytoma" of the parotid gland containing immunoglobulin crystals.

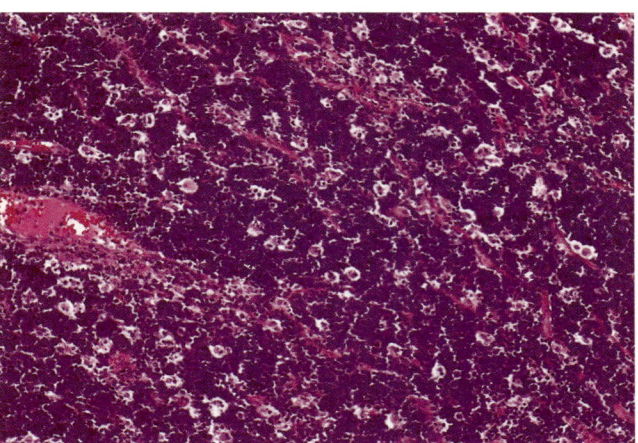

FIG. 11-35. Burkitt's lymphoma.

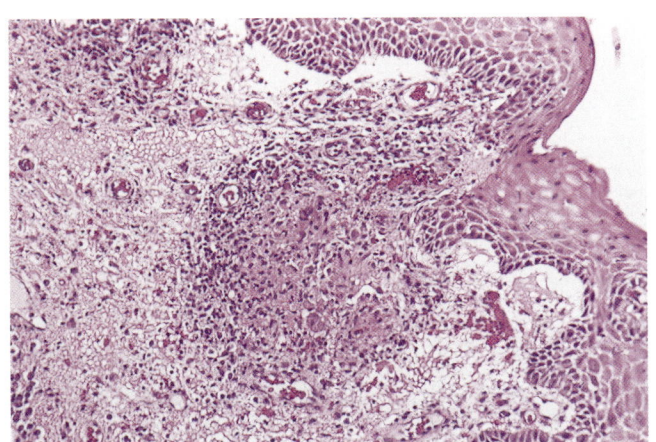

FIG. 11-36. Focal plasma cell granuloma.

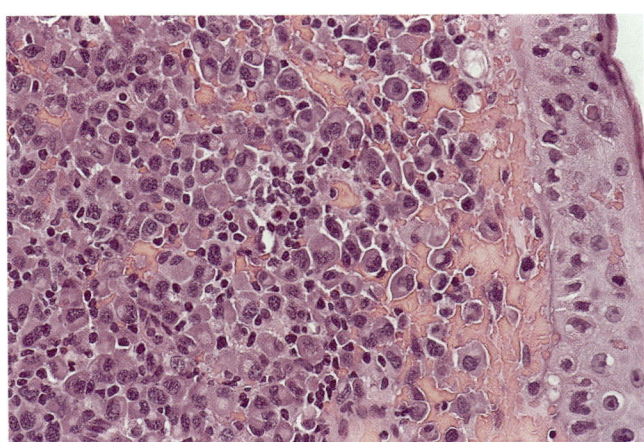

FIG. 11-37. Plasmacytoma.

LEIOMYOSARCOMA

Presentation

Leiomyosarcomas of the head and neck are quite rare. They generally present as an asymptomatic enlarging mass.

Pathophysiology

These tumors are usually solitary, slow-growing, painless masses.

Histology

Histologically, this is a cellular neoplasm composed of spindle-shaped cells that have elongated, centrally located, cigar-shaped nuclei with an eosinophilic cytoplasm. An infiltrative growth pattern and increased mitotic activity are hallmarks of this tumor. Leiomyomas, the benign counterpart, are composed of mature spindle-shaped cells and lack an infiltrative growth pattern and mitotic activity. Both the benign and malignant forms show immunoreactivity for smooth-muscle actin.

LIPOSARCOMA

Presentation

Liposarcomas generally present as slowly enlarging, asymptomatic masses. They are very rare in the head and neck.

Pathophysiology

Liposarcomas arise from lipoblasts or pleuripotential cells within or adjacent to fascial or intramuscular areas. They do not arise from a preexisting lipoma. In the head and neck, they are usually diagnosed when of a small size.

Histology

Liposarcomas can be divided into four subgroups: myxoid, round cell, well differentiated, and pleomorphic.

NEUROSARCOMA

Presentation

These tumors generally present as an expanding mass anywhere in the head and neck. Growth can be moderate to rapid. The tumors may also be associated with pain and paresthesias. They are generally firm, lobulated, and circumscribed.

Pathophysiology

For a diagnosis of primary neurogenous sarcoma to be made, it must be shown that the tumor arises from a nerve trunk. This is the only feature that distinguishes a neurogenous sarcoma from a fibrosarcoma.

Histology

Neurogenous sarcomas exhibit various patterns of pleomorphism of spindle-shaped cells. A cellular arrangement in strings or cords with tandem nuclei is a common finding. Most tumors are richly cellular and have conspicuous mitoses. The neoplastic spindled cells are often pleomorphic, with some having giant cell forms.

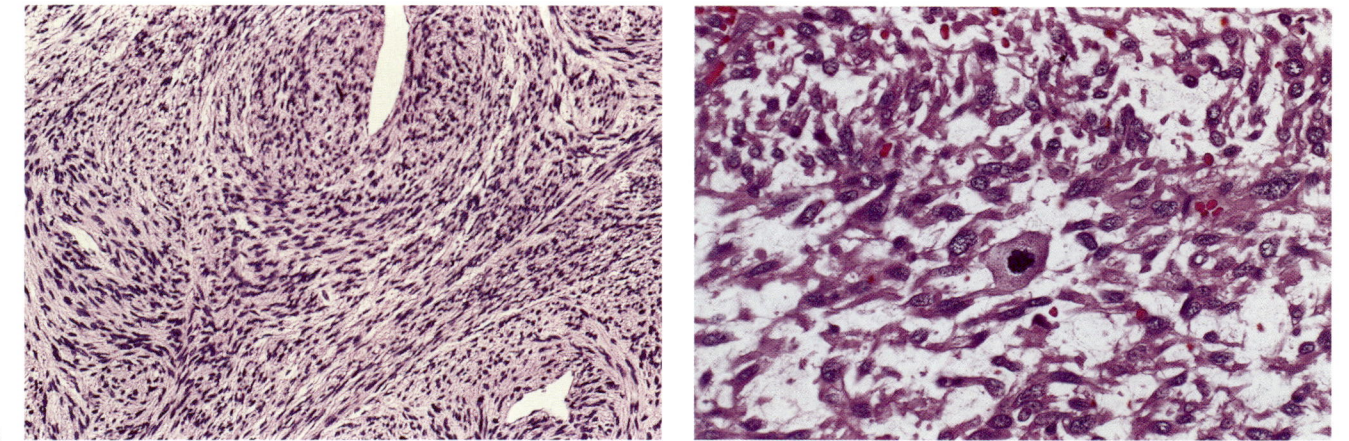

FIG. 11-38. A,B: Leiomyosarcomas in nasal cavity.

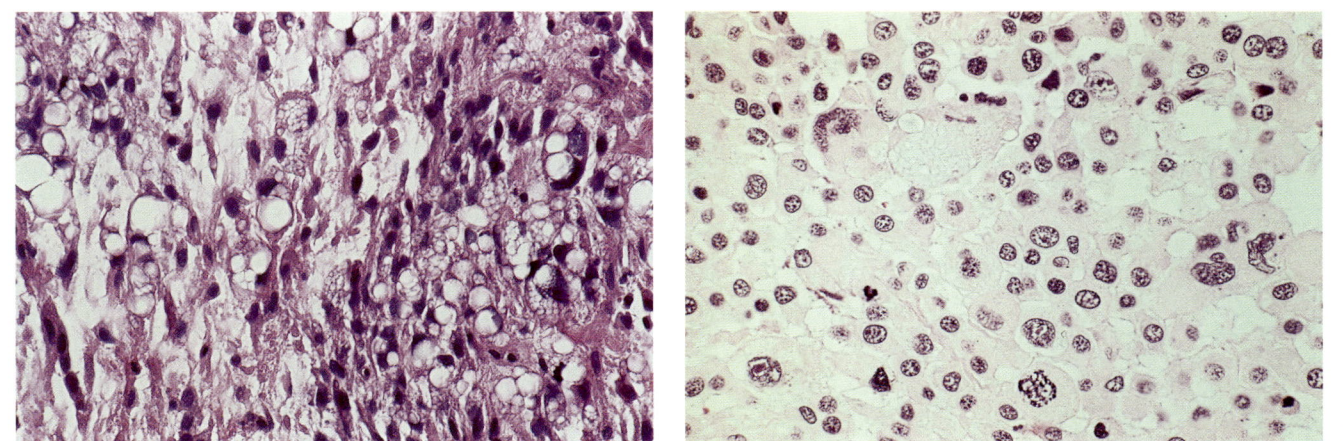

FIG. 11-39. A,B: Liposarcomas.

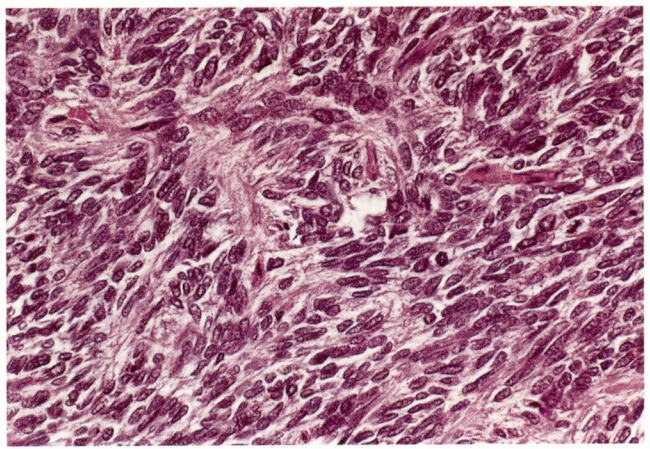

FIG. 11-40. Neurosarcoma. This neoplasm arose in a patient with von Recklinghausen's disease.

12

Noninflammatory, Nonneoplastic Diseases

FORDYCE'S GRANULES

Presentation

Fordyce's granules are usually noted on routine examination of the oral cavity.

Pathophysiology

Fordyce's granules consist of a collection of sebaceous glands within the oral cavity, often situated on the buccal mucosa. Lesions occur largely in adults, are present in approximately 80% of the normal adult population, and are generally asymptomatic. The gross appearance is that of small, yellow, raised spots.

Histology

Histologically, Fordyce's granules are shown to be sebaceous glands within the mucosa.

AMYLOIDOSIS

Presentation

The most common presenting symptom is hoarseness. In cases of laryngeal involvement, there is generally no systemic involvement.

Pathophysiology

Amyloidosis is characterized by the extracellular deposition of fibrillar protein, most commonly in the head and neck and involving either the larynx or the tongue. It is more common in men than in women and generally occurs in the fifth to sixth decade of life. In extralaryngeal sites, amyloidosis is often a manifestation of systemic disease.

Histology

In laryngeal amyloidosis, histology shows an extracellular eosinophilic amorphous material deposited throughout the submucosa. The epithelium is generally not involved. The material stains with Congo red or crystal violet, and apple green birefringence is seen under polarized light with the Congo red stain.

Chapter 12/Noninflammatory, Nonneoplastic Diseases

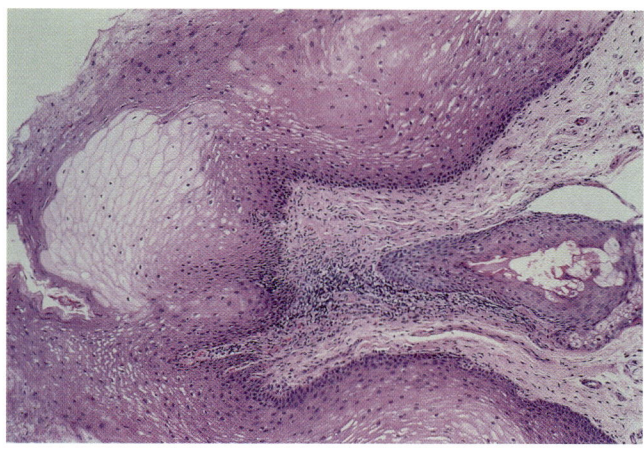

FIG. 12-1. Fordyce's granule.

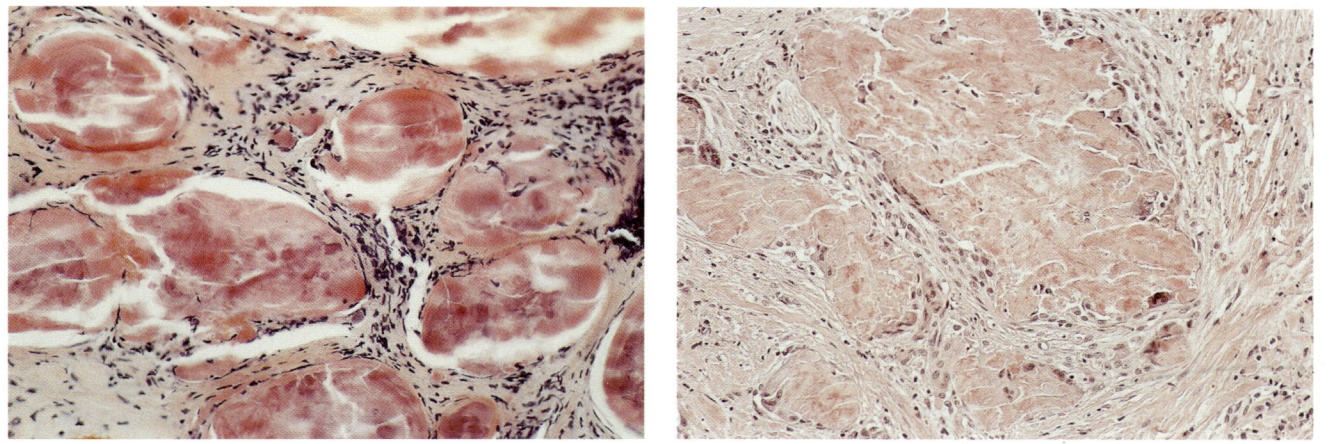

FIG. 12-2. A: Nodular amyloid deposits in larynx. **B:** Nodular amyloid deposits in parotid gland.

HEMANGIOMA

Presentation

Hemangiomas can occur anywhere on the body and anywhere in the head and neck. They are commonly cutaneous in and around the parotid gland and subglottic in the larynx. They generally develop in children and are usually apparent by the end of the first year of life.

Pathophysiology

Hemangiomas often show an early spurt of growth, but the vast majority involute by the time the patient is 5 or 6 years old. If they become obstructive in the subglottic region or do not involute in other areas, active treatment may be necessary.

Histology

Histologically, one sees an unencapsulated tumor with capillary-sized vessels lined by endothelial cells. Mitoses can be frequent.

LYMPHANGIOMA

Presentation

The general presentation is that of a soft, doughy, mobile mass, most commonly located in the neck.

Pathophysiology

Cystic hygromas presumably develop from portions of the lymphatic system that become separated from the primary lymphatic system during embryologic development. This is merely a special term for lymphangioma. Some prefer the term lymphatic malformation. Between 65% and 75% of cystic hygromas are diagnosed at or shortly after birth, and 85% appear within the first 3 years of life. The vast majority are found in the neck.

Histology

Histologically, the lesion is composed of large spaces lined by a single layer of endothelial cells and containing proteinaceous fluid with lymphocytes. There is a fibrous connective tissue stroma with occasional lymphoid aggregates.

Chapter 12/Noninflammatory, Nonneoplastic Diseases

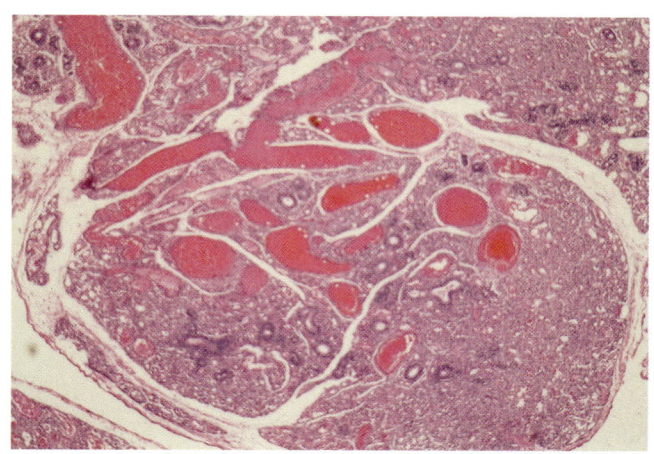
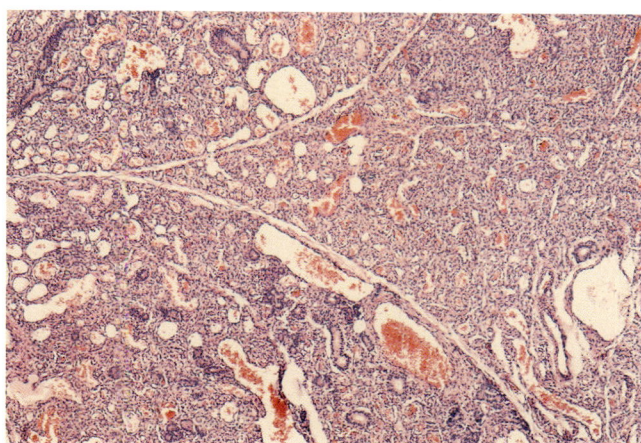

FIG. 12-3. A,B: Hemangioma of the parotid gland.

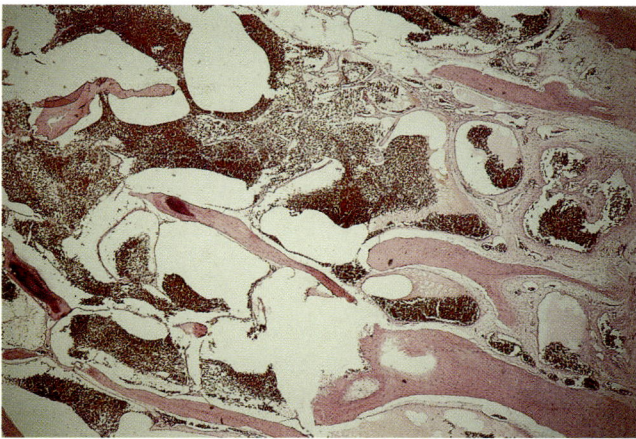

FIG. 12-4. Cavernous hemangioma of nasal bone.

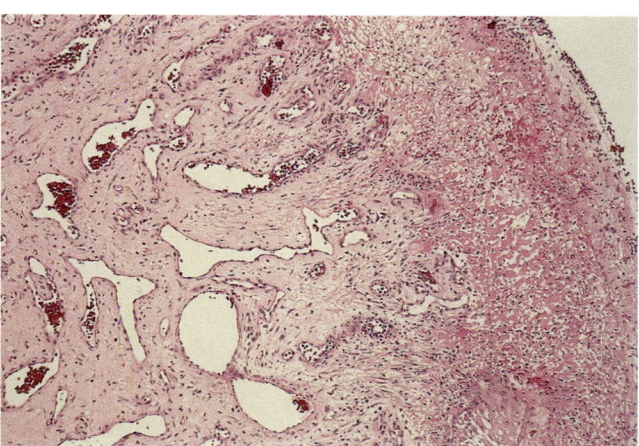

FIG. 12-5. Pyogenic granuloma in nasal cavity. This may be indistinguishable from a so-called "hemangioma of pregnancy."

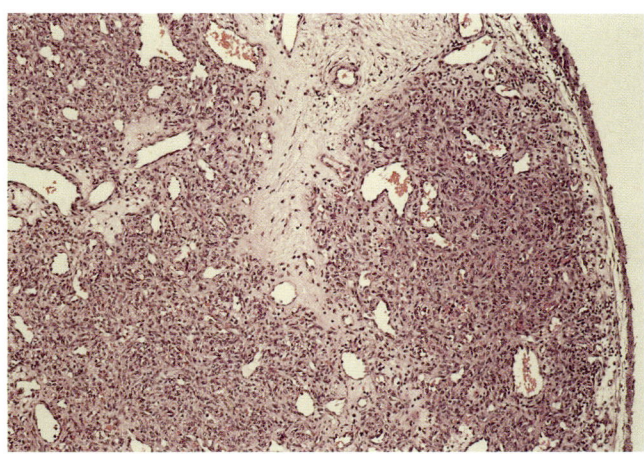

FIG. 12-6. Lobular hemangioma in nasal cavity.

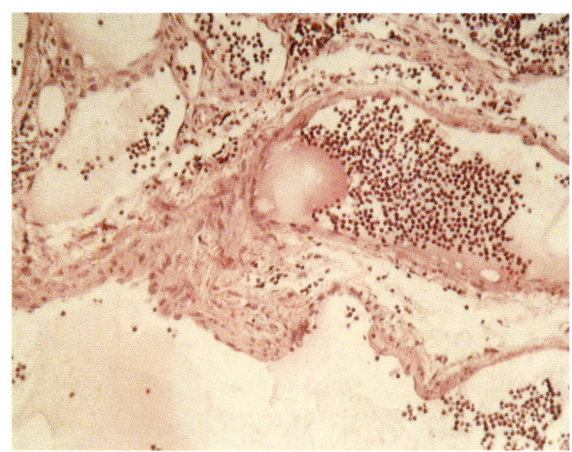

FIG. 12-7. Lymphangioma.

BRANCHIAL CLEFT CYST

Presentation

The cyst appears underneath the anterior edge of the sternocleidomastoid muscle at about the level of the hyoid bone or slightly below.

Pathophysiology

Ninety percent of branchial cleft cysts are felt to arise from the second arch, which connects internally with the tonsillar fossa and externally with the skin of the neck.

Histology

The cyst contains a clear to milky fluid, and the lining is usually squamous epithelium, although respiratory epithelium may be present. The lining epithelium is composed of stratified squamous cells or occasionally columnar epithelial cells. The cyst wall often contains a lymphoid infiltrate, occasionally with germinal centers.

Cysts of the first branchial cleft are much less common and can be subdivided into types I and II. Type I cysts are a duplication of the external auditory canal and contain only a squamous lining. Type II cysts are a duplication of ectoderm and mesoderm and typically contain cartilage as well. In any case, they are intimately associated with the facial nerve.

Chapter 12/Noninflammatory, Nonneoplastic Diseases

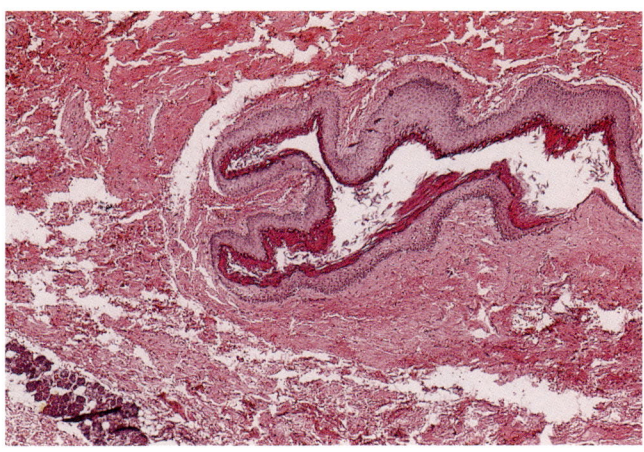

FIG. 12-8. First branchial cleft cyst.

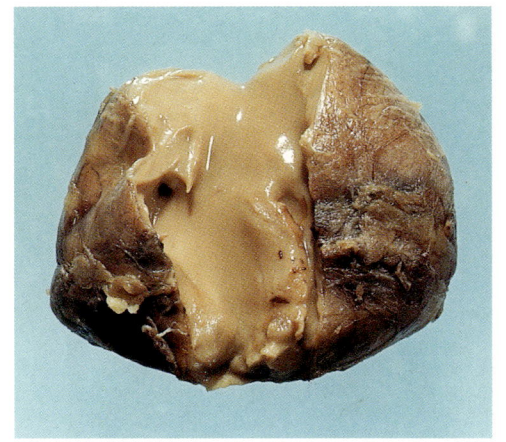

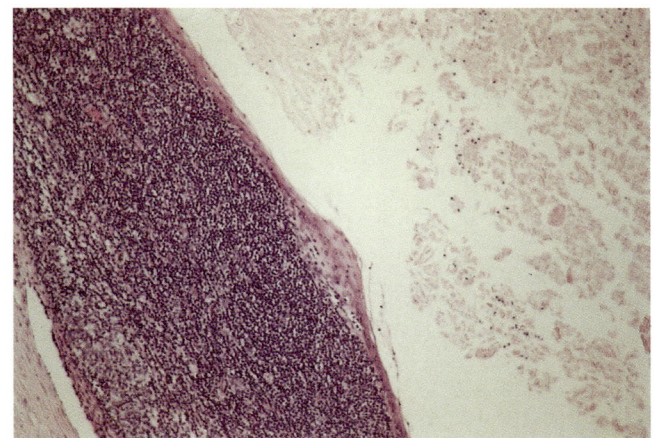

FIG. 12-9. Second branchial cleft cyst.

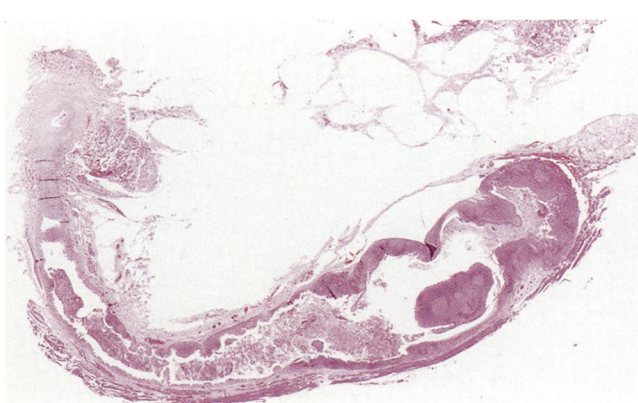

FIG. 12-10. A complete second branchial tract and cyst from pharyngeal mucosa to subcutaneous location.

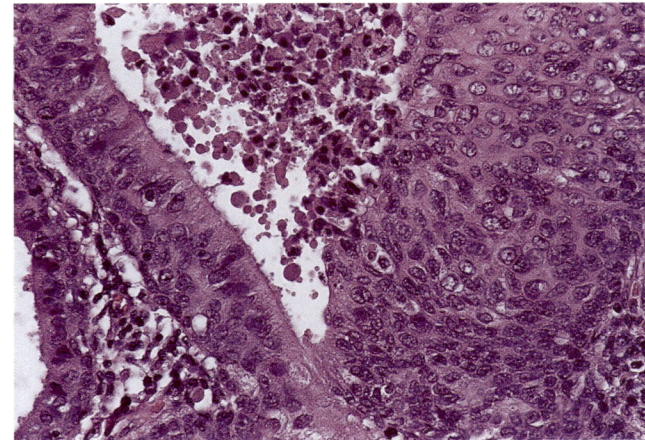

FIG. 12-11. A very rare primary branchiogenic carcinoma. Note the nonneoplastic epithelium with nonkeratinizing carcinoma originating from it.

NODULAR FASCIITIS

Presentation

Nodular fasciitis is a definite clinicopathologic entity and should not be classified under the general heading of fibromatosis. Nodular pseudosarcomatous fasciitis is most likely a reactive nonneoplastic response to injury. It generally presents as a tumorlike mass and is usually fast-growing.

Pathophysiology

The tumor is usually a discrete, soft-tissue mass that is somewhat tender and often fixed to subjacent structures, but with movable overlying skin. It is most likely a response to injury.

Histology

Histologically, one sees a haphazard arrangement of the regular bundles or single fibroblasts in a mucoid matrix. An important and constant feature is the vasculature of the lesion, which is composed of a fine capillary network arranged in a radial pattern. The predominant cells are large fibroblasts, and mitoses are common but never plentiful.

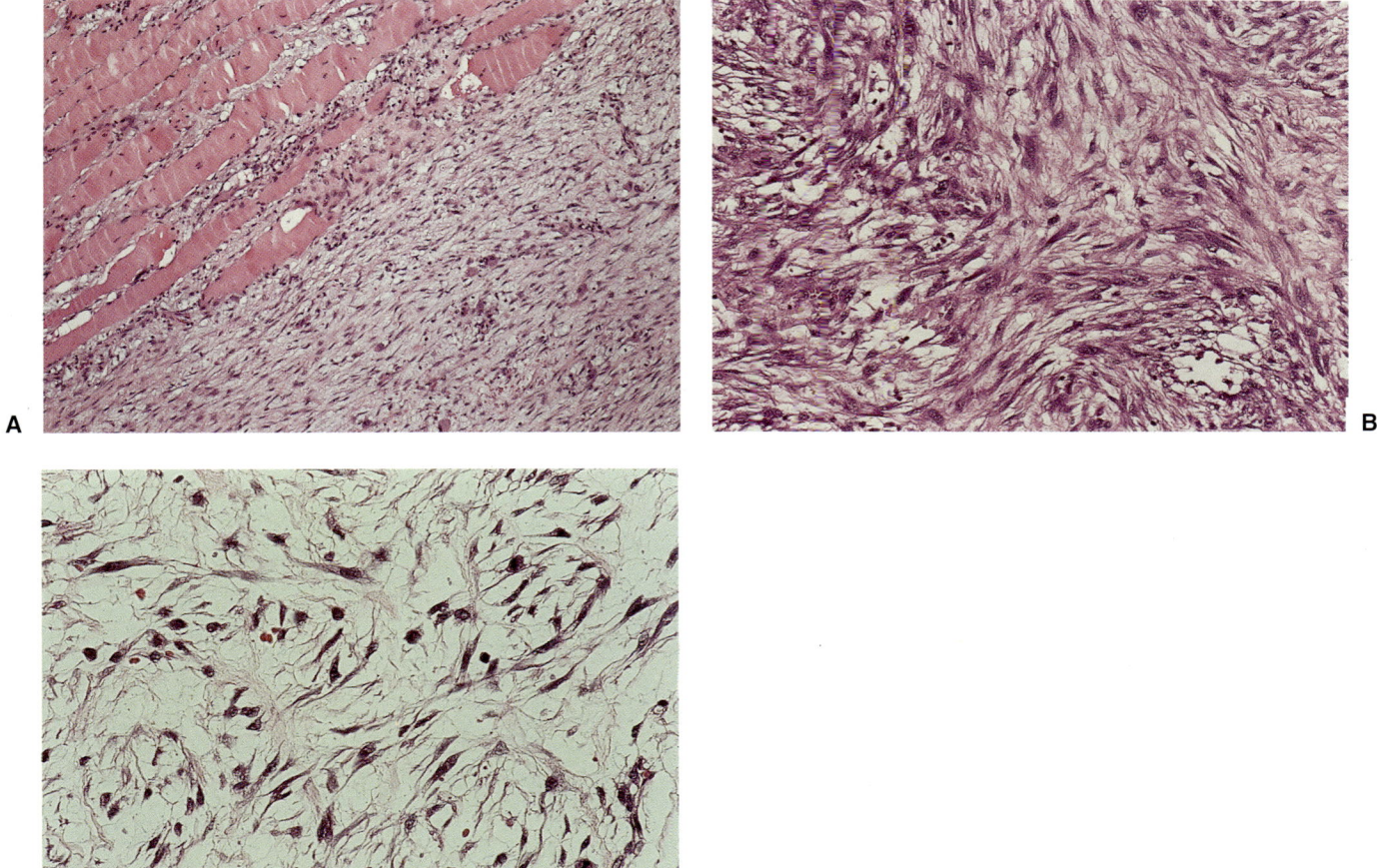

FIG 12-12. A–C: Nodular fasciitis.

Subject Index

Page numbers followed by "f" indicate figures; page numbers followed by "t" refer to tables.

A

Acinic cell adenocarcinoma
  clinical features of, 22
  cytologic features, 22, 22f–23f, 22t
  growth patterns, 22, 22t
  papillocystic, 23f
Actinic keratosis
  clinical presentation of, 90
  histology of, 90, 91f
  pathophysiology of, 90
Acute otitis media
  clinical presentation of, 66
  histology of, 66, 67f
  pathophysiology of, 66
Adenocarcinoma
  acinic cell
    clinical features of, 22
    growth patterns, 22, 22t
    histologic features, 22, 22f–23f, 22t
    papillocystic, 23f
  enteric, 84, 85f
  polymorphous low-grade
    clinical features of, 30
    differential diagnosis, 30
    histologic features of, 31f
    metastasis, 31f
  sinonasal
    clinical presentation of, 84
    histology of, 84, 85f
    pathophysiology of, 84
  of sinonasal tract, 84, 85f
  terminal duct
    clinical features of, 30
    differential diagnosis, 30
    histologic features of, 31f
    metastasis, 31f
Adenoid cystic carcinoma
  clinical course, 28
  cribriform, 28f
  cylindromatous, 28f
  high-grade, 29f
  histologic features of, 28f–29f
  metastatic, 29f
  perineural invasion, 28, 29f
  tubular, 28f
Adenomas
  basal cell
    clinical features of, 8
    growth patterns of, 8
    histologic features of, 9f
  canalicular
    clinical features of, 12
    histologic features of, 13f
  dermal analogue monomorphic, 16, 17f
  inverted ductal papilloma
    clinical features of, 12
    histologic features of, 14f
  middle ear, 67f
  myoepithelioma
    clear cell, 15f
    clinical features of, 14
    histologic features of, 14f–15f, 17f
  oncocytoma
    clinical features of, 10
    metaplasia, 11f, 13f
    of parotid gland, 10f–11f
  parathyroid, 60, 61f
  pleomorphic
    carcinoma ex, 24, 25f
    clinical features of, 6
    histologic features of, 7f
    metaplasia of, 6, 7f
    recurrent, 7f
    sebaceous, 19f
  Warthin's tumor
    clinical features of, 8
    cystic component of, 8, 9f
    histologic features of, 9f
    metaplasia of, 8
  WHO classification of, 5t
Adenomatoid odontogenic tumor
  clinical presentation of, 106
  histology of, 106, 107f
  pathophysiology of, 106
Adenomatous hyperplasia, 42
Albright's syndrome, 110
Allergic fungal sinusitis
  clinical presentation of, 78
  histology of, 78, 79f
  pathophysiology of, 78
Ameloblastoma
  clinical presentation of, 104
  histology of, 104, 105f
  pathophysiology of, 104
Amyloidosis
  clinical presentation of, 166
  histology of, 166, 167f
  laryngeal, 166, 167f
  pathophysiology of, 166

Anaplastic carcinoma
   histology of, 56, 57f
   pathophysiology of, 56
Aneurysmal bone cyst
   clinical presentation of, 114
   histology of, 114, 115f
   pathophysiology of, 114
Angiofibroma
   clinical presentation of, 82
   histology of, 82, 84
   pathophysiology of, 82

B

Basal cell adenoma
   clinical features of, 8
   growth patterns of, 8
   histologic features of, 9f
Basal cells, 4
B-cell lymphoma, 158, 159f–160f
Blastomyces dermatitidis, 132
Blastomycosis
   clinical presentation of, 132
   histologic findings of, 132, 133f
   pathophysiology of, 132
Branchial cleft cyst
   clinical presentation of, 170
   of first branchial cleft, 170, 171f
   histology of, 170, 171f
   pathophysiology of, 170
   of second branchial cleft, 170, 171f
Branchiogenic carcinoma, 171f
Burkitt's lymphoma, 161f

C

Canalicular adenoma
   clinical features of, 12
   histologic features of, 13f
   mucus secretions, 12
Candidiasis
   clinical presentation of, 98
   histology of, 98, 102f
   pathophysiology of, 98
Carcinoma. *See specific carcinoma*
Carcinoma *in situ,* 146
Cat-scratch disease
   clinical presentation of, 130
   histologic findings, 130, 131f
   pathophysiology of, 130
Cementifying fibroma, 112, 113f
Ceruminoma
   clinical presentation of, 64
   growth patterns of, 64
   histology of, 64
   pathophysiology of, 64
Cholesteatoma
   cholesterol granuloma and, 65f
   clinical presentation of, 64
   histology of, 64, 65f
   pathophysiology of, 64

Cholesterol granuloma
   cholesteatoma and, 65f
   clinical presentation of, 64
   histology of, 64, 65f
   pathophysiology of, 64
Chondroid chordoma, 125f
Chondroma
   clinical presentation of, 120
   of epiglottis, 121f
   histology of, 120, 121f
   pathophysiology of, 120
   of temporal bone, 121f
Chondromyxoid fibroma, 121f
Chondrosarcoma, 26
   clinical presentation of, 122
   histology of, 122, 123f
   in larynx, 122, 123f
   of maxilla, 123f
   myxoid, 123f
   pathophysiology of, 122
Chordoma
   chondroid, 125f
   clinical presentation of, 124
   histology of, 124, 125f
   pathophysiology of, 124
Choristoma, 116
Coccidioidomycosis
   clinical presentation of, 134
   histologic findings of, 134, 135f
   pathophysiology of, 134
Compound nevus, 90, 91f
Contact granuloma
   clinical presentation of, 72
   histology of, 72, 73f
   pathophysiology of, 72
Cyst
   aneurysmal bone
      clinical presentation of, 114
      histology of, 114, 115f
      pathophysiology of, 114
   branchial cleft
      clinical presentation of, 170
      of first branchial cleft, 170, 171f
      histology of, 170, 171f
      pathophysiology of, 170
      of second branchial cleft, 170, 171f
   thyroglossal duct, 48, 49f
Cystic hygroma. *See* Lymphangioma

D

Dermal analogue monomorphic adenoma, 16, 17f
Dermal analogue tumors, 8
Dermatofibrosarcoma
   clinical presentation of, 98
   histology of, 98, 99f
   pathophysiology of, 98
Disease. *See specific disease*

E

Endolymphatic sac tumors
   clinical presentation of, 68
   growth patterns, 68
   histology of, 68, 69f
   papillary, 69f
   pathophysiology of, 68
Enteric adenocarcinoma, 84, 85f
Eosinophilic granuloma
   clinical presentation of, 68
   histology of, 68, 69f
   pathophysiology of, 68
Epimyoepithelial carcinoma
   clinical features of, 32
   histologic features of, 33f
Erythroplakia, 146
External otitis, malignant
   clinical presentation of, 66
   histology of, 66, 67f
   pathophysiology of, 66

F

Fibroma
   cementifying, 112, 113f
   chondromyxoid, 121f
   odontogenic, 108, 109f
Fibromatosis
   clinical presentation of, 92
   desmoid, 92, 93f
   histology of, 92, 93f
   pathophysiology of, 92
Fibrosarcoma. *See also*
      Dermatofibrosarcoma
   clinical presentation of, 96
   histology of, 96, 97f
   pathophysiology of, 96
   types of, 96
Fibrotumefactive lesion, 97f
Fibrous dysplasia
   clinical presentation of, 110
   histology of, 110, 111f
   pathophysiology of, 110
   types of, 110
Fibrous tumors
   clinical presentation of, 92
   histology of, 92
   pathophysiology of, 92
Follicular carcinoma
   histology of, 52, 53f
   metastasis, 52
   pathophysiology of, 52
Fordyce's granules
   clinical presentation of, 166
   histology of, 166, 167f
   pathophysiology of, 166
Fungiform papilloma
   clinical presentation of, 82
   histology of, 82, 83f
   pathophysiology of, 82

G

Gardner's syndrome, 116
Giant cell granuloma
  clinical presentation of, 114
  histology of, 114, 115f
  pathophysiology of, 114
Goiter
  anaplastic carcinoma and, 56
  multinodular, 48, 49f
Granular cell tumor
  clinical presentation of, 138
  histology of, 138
  pathophysiology of, 138
Granuloma
  cholesterol
    cholesteatoma and, 65f
    clinical presentation of, 64
    histology of, 64, 65f
    pathophysiology of, 64
  contact
    clinical presentation of, 72
    histology of, 72, 73f
    pathophysiology of, 72
  eosinophilic
    clinical presentation of, 68
    histology of, 68, 69f
    pathophysiology of, 68
  giant cell
    clinical presentation of, 114
    histology of, 114, 115f
    pathophysiology of, 114
  pyogenic, 169f
Graves' disease, 48, 49f

H

Hand-Schüller-Christian disease, 68
Hashimoto's thyroiditis, 48, 49f
Hemangioma
  cavernous, 169f
  clinical presentation of, 168
  histology of, 168, 169f
  lobular, 169f
  pathophysiology of, 168
Herpes simplex virus
  clinical presentation of, 98
  histology of, 98, 102f
  pathophysiology of, 98
Hibernoma
  clinical presentation of, 140
  histology of, 140, 141f
  pathophysiology of, 140
Histiocytosis X, 68
Human immunodeficiency virus
  lymphoepithelial lesions in, 38f
  mucormycosis in, 78, 79f
Hürthle cell carcinoma
  histology of, 54, 55f
  pathophysiology of, 54
Hygroma. See Lymphangioma

Hyperkeratosis, 146
Hyperparathyroidism
  clinical presentation of, 60
  histology of, 60, 61f
  pathophysiology of, 60

I

Inflammatory pseudotumor, 97f
Intradermal nevus, 90, 91f
Inverted ductal papilloma
  clinical features of, 12
  histologic features of, 14f
Inverted papilloma
  clinical presentation of, 82
  histology of, 82, 83f
  pathophysiology of, 82
  squamous cell carcinoma and, 82

J

Junctional nevus, 90, 91f

K

Keloids
  clinical presentation of, 94
  histology of, 94, 95f
  pathophysiology of, 94
Klebsiella rhinoscleromatis, 130, 131f. *See also* Rhinoscleroma
Küttner tumor, 44, 45f

L

Langerhans cell histiocytosis, 68
Langerhans' giant cells, 134
Leiomyoma
  clinical presentation of, 140
  histology of, 140, 141f
  pathophysiology of, 140
Leiomyosarcoma
  clinical presentation of, 162
  histology of, 162, 163f
  pathophysiology of, 162
Leprosy
  clinical presentation of, 132
  histologic findings of, 132, 133f
  lepromatous, 132
  perineural granuloma associated with, 133f
  tuberculoid, 132
Letterer-Siwe syndrome, 68
Lindsay tumor, 54, 55f
Lingual osteoma, 117f
Lingual thyroid, 48
Lipoma
  clinical presentation of, 140
  histology of, 140, 141f
  pathophysiology of, 140
Liposarcoma

  clinical presentation of, 162
  histology of, 162, 163f
  pathophysiology of, 162
Lymphadenitis
  granulomatous, 135f
  toxoplasmosis, 134, 135f
Lymphadenoma
  sebaceous, 19f
Lymphangioma
  clinical presentation of, 168
  histology of, 168, 169f
  pathophysiology of, 168
Lymphoepithelial lesions, relation to Sjögren's syndrome
  description of, 36
  follicular lymphoid hyperplasia associated with, 38f
  histologic features of, 37f–39f
  in HIV-infected patients, 38f
Lymphoma
  B-cell, 158, 159f
  Burkitt's, 161f
  clinical presentation of, 158
  histology of, 158
  nasal, 160f
  non-Hodgkin's, 158, 159f
  pathophysiology of, 158
  Sjögren's syndrome and, 158

M

Malignant external otitis
  clinical presentation of, 66
  histology of, 66, 67f
  pathophysiology of, 66
Malignant mixed tumor
  benign metastasizing, 24, 24f
  carcinoma ex pleomorphic adenoma
    clinical features of, 24t
    histologic features of, 25f
    metastatic, 25f
  description of, 22
  sarcomatoid, 26, 27f
  true, 26, 27f
MALT. *See* Mucosa-associated lymphoid tissue
Medullary carcinoma
  familial, 56
  histology of, 56, 57f
  pathophysiology of, 56
  sporadic, 56
Melanoma
  clear cell, 101f
  clinical presentation of, 98
  histology of, 98, 99f
  malignant, 100f
  metastasis of, 101f
  mucosal, 99f–100f
  pathophysiology of, 98
  superficial spreading, 99f

MEN. *See* Multiple endocrine neoplasia
Mikulicz's cells, 130, 131f
Mole. *See* Nevus
Monomorphic adenomas. *See* Basal cell adenoma
Mucocele
  anatomic predilection, 40
  clinical features of, 40
  histologic features of, 41f
Mucoepidermoid carcinoma
  clinical features of, 20, 22
  epidermoid cells, 20
  histologic features of, 20f–21f
  intermediate, 21f
  metastatic, 21f
  mucous cells, 20
  squamous cell carcinoma and, differential diagnosis between, 22
Mucormycosis
  clinical presentation of, 78
  histology of, 78, 79f
  pathophysiology of, 78
Mucosa-associated lymphoid tissue
  B-cell lymphoma of, 160f
  description of, 36
Multinodular goiter, 48, 49f
Multiple endocrine neoplasia, 56
Mycobacterial infections
  clinical presentation of, 130
  histology of, 130
  pathophysiology of, 130
Mycobacterium spp.
  M. leprae, 132, 133f
  M. tuberculosis, 130
Myoepithelial cells
  of salivary glands, 4
Myoepithelioma
  clear cell, 15f
  clinical features of, 14
  histologic features of, 14f–15f, 17f
Myofibroblastic tumor, 97f
Myospherulosis
  clinical presentation of, 80
  histology of, 80, 81f
  pathophysiology of, 80
Myxoma
  clinical presentation of, 114
  histology of, 114, 115f
  odontogenic
    clinical presentation of, 108
    dental pulp and, differentiation between, 109f
    histology of, 108, 109f
    pathophysiology of, 108
  pathophysiology of, 114

N

Nasal polyps
  angiomatous, 77f
  clinical presentation of, 76
  histology of, 76, 77f
  pathophysiology of, 76
Necrotizing external otitis. *See* Malignant external otitis
Necrotizing sialometaplasia
  clinical features of, 42
  histologic features of, 43f
Neuroblastoma
  olfactory
    clinical presentation of, 86
    grading system for, 86
    histology of, 86, 87f
    pathophysiology of, 86
Neurofibroma
  cutaneous, 139f
  plexiform, 139f
Neurosarcoma
  clinical presentation of, 162
  histology of, 162, 163f
  pathophysiology of, 162
Nevus
  compound, 90, 91f
  intradermal, 90, 91f
  junctional, 90, 91f
Nodular fasciitis
  clinical presentation of, 172
  histology of, 172, 173
  pathophysiology of, 172
Non-Hodgkin's lymphoma. *See* Lymphoma

O

Odontogenic fibroma, 108, 109f
Odontogenic keratocyst
  clinical presentation of, 104
  histology of, 104, 105f
  pathophysiology of, 104
Odontogenic myxoma
  clinical presentation of, 108
  dental pulp and, differentiation between, 109f
  histology of, 108, 109f
  pathophysiology of, 108
Odontogenic tumors
  adenomatoid
    clinical presentation of, 106
    histology of, 106, 107f
    pathophysiology of, 106
  clear cell, 107f
  squamous
    clinical presentation of, 106
    histology of, 106, 107f
    pathophysiology of, 106
Olfactory neuroblastoma
  clinical presentation of, 86
  grading system for, 86
  histology of, 86, 87f
  pathophysiology of, 86
Oncocyte cells, 10, 10f
Oncocytoma
  clinical features of, 10
  metaplasia, 11f, 13f
  of parotid gland, 10f–11f
Ossifying fibroma
  clinical presentation of, 112
  histology of, 112, 113f
  pathophysiology of, 112
Osteoblastoma
  clinical presentation of, 110
  histology of, 110, 111f
  pathophysiology of, 110
Osteochondroma
  clinical presentation of, 116
  histology of, 116, 117f
  pathophysiology of, 116
Osteoid osteoma
  clinical presentation of, 110
  histology of, 110, 111f
  pathophysiology of, 110
Osteoma
  clinical presentation of, 116
  histology of, 116, 117f
  osteoid. *See* Osteoid osteoma
  pathophysiology of, 116
Osteosarcoma
  clinical presentation of, 118
  histology of, 118, 119f
  pathophysiology of, 118
Otitis externa, malignant
  clinical presentation of, 66
  histology of, 66, 67f
  pathophysiology of, 66
Otitis media, acute
  clinical presentation of, 66
  histology of, 66, 67f
  pathophysiology of, 66

P

Paget's disease
  clinical presentation of, 124
  histology of, 124, 125f
  pathophysiology of, 124
Palate
  terminal duct adenocarcinoma of, 31f
Paneth's cell metaplasia, 85f
Papillary fronds, 8
Papillary thyroid carcinoma
  clinical features of, 50
  follicular variant of, 54, 55f
  histologic features of, 51f
  metastatic, 51f
Papilloma
  fungiform
    clinical presentation of, 82
    histology of, 82, 83f
    pathophysiology of, 82
  inverted
    clinical presentation of, 82
    histology of, 82, 83f

pathophysiology of, 82
squamous cell carcinoma and, 82
inverted ductal
clinical features of, 12
histologic features of, 14f
squamous
clinical presentation of, 72
histology of, 72, 73f
pathophysiology of, 72
Paraganglioma
carotid body, 142f–143f
clinical presentation of, 142
histology of, 142f–143f
pathophysiology of, 142
vagal body, 143f
Parathyroid gland
adenoma, 60, 61f
carcinoma of
clinical presentation of, 60
fibrosis associated with, 61f
histology of, 60, 61f
pathophysiology of, 60
pleomorphism associated with, 61f
normal histologic appearance of, 61f
Parotid gland. See also Salivary glands
amyloidosis of, 167f
anatomy of, 4
benign tumors of
dermal analogue monomorphic
adenoma, 17f
lipoma, 141f
oncocytoma, 10f–11f
pleomorphic adenoma, 7f
plexiform neurofibroma, 139f
hemangioma of, 169f
lymphoepithelial lesion of, 37f, 39f
malignancies of
acinic cell adenocarcinoma, 22f
adenoid cystic carcinoma, 28f
carcinoma ex pleomorphic adenoma, 22f
epimyoepithelial carcinoma, 33f
neuroendocrine carcinoma, 39f
non-Hodgkin's lymphoma, 159f
salivary duct carcinoma, 35f
sarcomatoid, 27f
melanoma metastasis to, 101f
sialadenitis of, 45f
in Sjögren's syndrome patients, 40
Pindborg tumor
clinical presentation of, 106
histology of, 106, 107f
pathophysiology of, 106
Plasmacytoma
clinical presentation of, 158
histology of, 158, 161f
pathophysiology of, 158
recurrences, 158
Pleomorphic adenoma
carcinoma ex, 24, 25f
clinical features of, 6

histologic features of, 7f
metaplasia of, 6, 7f
recurrent, 7f
Polymorphous low-grade adenocarcinoma
clinical features of, 30
differential diagnosis, 30
histologic features of, 31f
metastasis, 31f
Polyps. See Nasal polyps
Pseudomonas aeruginosa, 66
Pyogenic granuloma, 169f

R

Ranula
anatomic predilection, 40
clinical features of, 40
histologic features of, 41f
plunging, 40, 41f
Rhabdomyoma
adult type, 141f
clinical presentation of, 140
histology of, 140, 141f
infantile type, 141f
pathophysiology of, 140
Rhabdomyosarcoma
alveolar, 156, 157f
clinical presentation of, 156
embryonal, 156, 157f
histology of, 156, 157f
pathophysiology of, 156
Rhinoscleroma
clinical presentation of, 130
histologic findings of, 130, 131f
Mikulicz's cells, 130, 131f
pathophysiology of, 130
Rhinosporidiosis
clinical presentation of, 132
histologic findings of, 132, 133f
pathophysiology of, 132

S

Salivary duct carcinoma
clinical features of, 34
facial nerve branch invasion by, 35f
histologic features of, 35f
Salivary glands. See also specific salivary
gland
anatomy of, 4
benign tumors
basal cell adenoma, 8, 9f
canalicular adenoma, 12, 13f
classification of, 5t
dermal analogue monomorphic
adenoma, 6, 7f
histogenesis of, 4
inverted ductal papilloma, 12, 14f
myoepithelioma, 14, 14f–15f
oncocytoma, 10, 10f–11f
pleomorphic adenoma, 6, 7f

sebaceous tumors, 18, 19f
sialoblastoma, 18, 18f
Warthin's tumor, 8, 9f
lymph nodes in, 4
malignant tumors
acinic cell adenocarcinoma, 22, 22f–23f
adenoid cystic carcinoma, 28, 28f–29f
epimyoepithelial carcinoma, 32, 33f
malignant mixed tumor. See
Malignant mixed tumor
morphology of, 20
mucoepidermoid carcinoma, 20f–21f, 20–22
polymorphous low-grade
adenocarcinoma, 30, 31f
salivary duct carcinoma, 34, 35f
nonneoplastic lesions of
lymphoepithelial lesions, relation to
Sjögren's syndrome, 36, 37f–39f, 40
mucocele, 40
necrotizing sialometaplasia, 42, 43f
ranula, 40
sialadenitis, 44, 45f
sialolithiasis, 42, 43f
sialosis, 36, 36f
Sarcoidosis
clinical presentation of, 134
histologic findings of, 134, 135f
noncaseating granulomas of, 134, 135f
pathophysiology of, 134
Sarcoma. See specific sarcoma
Sarcomatoid, 26, 27f
Sarcomatoid carcinoma, 150, 153f–154f
Schneiderian papilloma.
Schwannoma
Antoni A areas, 138, 139f
clinical presentation of, 138
histology of, 138, 139f
pathophysiology of, 138
Sebaceous tumors, 18, 19f
Seborrheic keratosis
clinical presentation of, 92
histology of, 92, 93f
pathophysiology of, 92
Sialadenitis
clinical features of, 44
histologic features of, 45f
Sialadenosis, 36
Sialoblastoma, 18, 18f
Sialolithiasis, 42, 43f
Sialometaplasia, necrotizing
clinical features of, 42
histologic features of, 43f
Sialosis, 36, 36f
Sinonasal adenocarcinoma
clinical presentation of, 84
histology of, 84, 85f
pathophysiology of, 84

Sinusitis, allergic fungal
  clinical presentation of, 78
  histology of, 78, 79f
  pathophysiology of, 78
Sjögren's syndrome
  clinical presentation, 40
  histology, 40
  lymphoepithelial lesions associated with
    description of, 36
    follicular lymphoid hyperplasia
      associated with, 38f
    histologic features of, 37f–39f
    in HIV-infected patients, 38f
  lymphoma and, 158
Solitary fibrous tumors, 97f
Squamous cell carcinoma
  adenoid, 147f
  basaloid, 148f, 150
  clinical presentation of, 146
  histology of, 146, 146f–149f
  invasive, 147f
  inverted papilloma and, 82
  metastatic, 149f, 155f
  mucoepidermoid carcinoma and,
    differential diagnosis between, 22
  nonkeratinizing, 147f, 150
  overview of, 150
  papillary, 150, 152f
  pathophysiology of, 146
  risk factors, 146
  sarcomatoid, 150, 153f–154f
  verrucous carcinoma and, differentiation
    between, 150, 151f–152f
Squamous odontogenic tumor
  clinical presentation of, 106
  histology of, 106, 107f
  pathophysiology of, 106
Squamous papilloma
  clinical presentation of, 72
  histology of, 72, 73f
  pathophysiology of, 72
Sublingual gland
  anatomy of, 4
  ranula of, 40
Submandibular gland
  anatomy of, 4
  Küttner tumor of, 44
  sialadenitis of, 45f
Syndromes. *See specific syndrome*

T
Terminal duct adenocarcinoma
  clinical features of, 30
  differential diagnosis, 30
  histologic features of, 31f
  metastasis, 31f
Thyroglossal duct cyst, 48, 49f
Toxoplasma gondii, 134
Toxoplasmosis
  clinical presentation of, 134
  histologic findings of, 134, 135f
  lymphadenitis, 134, 135f
  pathophysiology of, 134
Tumor. *See specific tumor*

V
Verocay bodies, 138
Verrucous carcinoma
  description of, 150
  squamous cell carcinoma and,
    differentiation between, 150,
    151f–152f
Vocal fold nodules
  clinical presentation of, 72
  histology of, 72, 73f
  pathophysiology of, 72
von Hippel-Lindau disease, 68

W
Warthin's tumor
  clinical features of, 8
  cystic component of, 8, 9f
  histologic features of, 9f
  metaplasia of, 8
Wegener's granulomatosis
  clinical presentation of, 80
  histology of, 80, 81f
  pathophysiology of, 80
  vasculitis findings associated with, 81f